Untangling Alzheimer's

Untangling Alzheimer's

The Guide for Families and Professionals

TAM CUMMINGS, PHD

Library of Congress Control Number: 2013936678
CreateSpace Independent Publishing Platform
North Charleston, South Carolina

Cummings, Tam, 1961-
Untangling Alzheimer's: The Guide for Families and Professionals/ Tam Cummings – 2nd
edition

ISBN: 0990963713
ISBN 978-0-9909637-1-4 (softcover)

1. Dementia. 2. Alzheimer's Disease. 3. Health Education. 4. Aging.
5. Mental Health

Second Edition
10 9 8 7 6 5 4 3

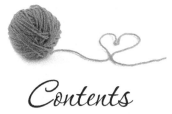

Contents

To my mother
Margie L. Cummings
who taught me this:

"And now abideth faith,
hope and charity, these three,
but the greatest of these is charity."
1 Corinthians 13:13, KJV

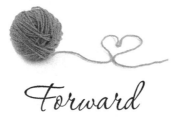

Forward

Untangling Alzheimer's is a very welcome addition to information available to the public, healthcare providers and especially caregivers on disorders of the brain that leave the individual cognitively and physically impaired and requiring full-time care.

Tam Cummings uses her extensive experience in dementia to take the reader, at a very personal level, along the path of observation and caring, in a way that makes a complex disease and the role it plays in the lives of the individual, family, caregivers and friends, much more understandable.

Although ***Untangling Alzheimer's*** is predominantly focused on Dementia of the Alzheimer's Type, it provides the necessary information to understand the very similar mental and physical declines found in many other forms of dementia.

The book is easy to read and provides very valuable information, along with case examples of the various stages of cognitive and personality decline that inevitably occur in dementia. It especially provides very useful tips for the reader on behavior and communication problems that commonly occur in dementia and suggests different ways to cope and adjust for them.

The section on "dying" is very special, because it describes the last stages of dementia in a very humane and informative way so that the readers feel that their loved one has been treated and cared for in the best possible manner and will now "rest in peace."

Tam does a superb job in ***Untangling Alzheimer's*** with her personal skill, experience and caring dialogue. It makes it seem as though she is in the room with the reader. This book is a must read for those who know or care for a person with dementia.

Ronald Devere, MD, FAAN

Board Certified Neurologist

Director, Alzheimer's Disease and Memory Disorders Center

Austin, Texas

Acknowledgment

I would like to thank the friends and colleagues who have provided support and guidance throughout the process of producing this book. Ronald Devere, M.D. and Dennis Myers, Ph.D., are two gifted men who continue to teach and mentor me.

My friends and colleagues: Carla Cochran, RN, CALM, Susan Frederickson, Terria Jones, CALM, Diane McKinnon and Glenda Rodgers, provided input and critical feedback as professionals who work every day with family and professional caregivers and persons diagnosed with dementia.

Mary and Key Norris, Frank and Sally Martin, John Turner, Mary LaTouf, Pat Cutrone, Robyn Seiferth, Heidi Green and Helen Hooper: as family caregivers you offered me insights into your loved ones' lives and helped me grow as a professional. Thanks to you all.

To my spouse Lt. Col. Tammy L. Knott, (U.S. Army Retired) your love and support allows me to help so many families and professionals.

Edited by Erin Dewald.

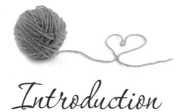

Introduction

The information and stories in this book are designed to take the fear and mystery out of a dementia diagnosis and explain a complex disease process in a way that will make sense to a family or professional caregiver. The first two chapters will describe the overall picture and history of dementia and Alzheimer's disease, the most common form of dementia. Additional chapters will explain how specific behaviors are a result of the disease impacting the brain, rather than a deliberate action or choice by the person with the disease. The content of this book will help guide you through the dementia process and explain the disease from the diagnosis to death and hopefully assist you in being the best caregiver possible.

The contents will also walk you through the stages of the disease, allowing you to identify the behaviors and changes as they are related to brain damage in the four lobes of the brain. It will cover specific techniques you can use to communicate and work with persons who have a dementia diagnosis, including how to approach, talk to, or provide activities for your loved one. And finally, it will explain the changes in the body during the final year of life and explore what feelings you can expect as a family member as you grieve for your loved one.

As we go forward in this book, I will use the feminine forms of words (e.g., she, her, mom) to avoid confusion. This is not to suggest women are at a higher risk for dementia than men. We see more female dementia patients than males because women statistically outlive men. Since women live longer, more women will develop dementia in some form. At the same time, some forms of dementias may be found more often in males, such as CADASIL, Lewy Bodies Dementia or Behavioral Variant Frontal Temporal Dementia. Otherwise, dementias affect about the same percentages in both sexes.

I fully recognize not everyone is dealing with an ill parent. Many of you are caregivers of spouses or siblings or neighbors or are court-appointed guardians or case managers. The experience for each of you will be different because of the varied emotions that come with each relationship, so please do not be offended by the use of the feminine noun.

As a family caregiver, whether you are the spouse, child, parent or friend who will be overseeing or providing care, you may experience denial, grief, guilt, anger and a host of other normal emotions. Dementia, in any of its forms, means the aging process for your loved one has changed dramatically, and so will your relationship.

The challenges you will face as a caregiver may feel staggering at times. Your efforts to provide care for your person at home can mean you may be frequently frustrated, angry, depressed and/or exhausted, often all at the same time. Odds are that by the time you seek outside care (typically about Stage Five), you will be in worse physical and emotional shape than your loved one.

By learning how this disease is affecting your loved one, you may be able to take some of the hurt out of the behaviors, and you will hopefully be able to experience a successful day or hour on this long journey. You will also have a greater chance of lowering your stress by learning about and understanding the disease.

Finally, keep in mind that many of you may find the information in this book difficult to read as you recognize scenarios and behaviors you see in your loved one. If you find yourself getting upset, simply set the book aside and come back to it later. Just know that once you understand what this disease is doing to the brain of the person you love and how that damage changes your loved one physically and emotionally, you will be a better caregiver. And hopefully, you will be more prepared and patient as you face the final journey of your loved one's life.

Up to this point, you have been doing the best you can as a caregiver with what you knew about the disease. But now you'll know what dementia is doing to the brain and, as a result, why your mom asks the same question over and over, why she confuses you with someone else, why bathing can be an issue and why she is "Sun downing."

Finally, I am sorry this disease has struck someone you love, for dementia is a cruel and unmatched disease. It takes away part of your heart as it destroys the brain and body of your loved one. Take a deep breath for you are not alone.

I wish you all the best,

Tam

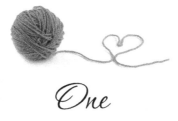

One

An Introduction to Dementia

In order for you as a professional or family member to be able to provide quality care for a person with dementia, you have to know and understand what the disease will do to her brain. Recognizing that the behaviors you may have already witnessed are a result of damage caused to the brain by the disease can greatly reduce your stress as a caregiver.

Knowing what dementia means, what the diseases of dementia are, and finally how the disease starts, its progression and impact on the brain, are the keys to providing care. Everything your loved one is doing is being driven by what's happening in her brain.

This book is designed to be a tool to allow you to know what dementia is and understand the difference between dementia and Alzheimer's (the most common form of dementia). Understanding the disease process will take the fear and confusion out of the behaviors your loved one exhibits. Reducing your own stress means you are a better caregiver, your own health is less at risk, and you are prepared for the changes your loved one will undergo as the disease progresses.

The word "dementia" is an umbrella term that means we are talking about one of an identified 48 forms of diseases in the brain. In order for a person to have one or more of these dementias, the disease process must affect at least two of the four lobes of the brain. Since the brain controls all memory and body function, it helps to understand that memory is what allows each of us to navigate our way through each day.

Let's start with a brief review of memory.

What Memory Means

Memory is not just who I am as a person or where I am going this afternoon. It is the ability to understand where I am, who I am, how to move muscles, how to recognize loved ones, how to use items around the house or at work. Memory is what has happened in the past and how the lessons learned from the past will affect how I act or approach problems in the future.

This can be as simple as learning and then remembering what the sound of a warning buzzer indicates. A buzzer in the home can mean the microwave went off, or that it is time to move clothes from the washing machine to the dryer.

Or a warning buzzer can indicate smoke has been detected, smoke means fire, and fire means danger. Memory and the use of memory tells you if the smoke is burning toast or a burning house. Is the smoke from a barbecue in the neighborhood or is the food on the stove on fire and there is an imminent threat to your safety?

Memory is what we have built on from infancy through today; it is what allows us to make sense of our world, both at home and at large. It is what we see and how we translate what we are seeing. Memory is how we interpret signals from our body and how we understand the stimuli around us. Memory is everything you can do or learn to do.

Our memories begin at the moment of birth. From the instant we are born, people are talking to us, welcoming us to the world. Introductions begin immediately, "I'm your momma," or "I'm your daddy," or "Say hello to grandpa."

Memories begin in infancy and continue to be added to throughout life. They are the building blocks by which we learn language and its nuances. Memory is what allows us to know and understand the steps it takes to complete the thousand variations of our every day tasks. Memory is how we interpret signals from our body. Memory allows you to hold your head up. Memories give us the ability to move muscles, recognize our loved ones and old friends. Memories and our interpretation of the experiences they represent, are what make each of us unique.

Losing your memory means losing the ability to do all the things we must do throughout each day and night. Loss of memory isn't just forgetting items on the shopping list, or the name of your spouse or child. It is the loss of everything we see and know and react to around us. Losing memory means losing how you understand your environment, or how you speak, walk, or care for yourself. Memory is everything we do as humans. It is how we get from point A to point B. Memory allows us to know who, what, where, when, why and how.

"She's Going to Lose Her Memory."

Let's try something we do every day that seems relatively simple, but requires a great many steps of memory. We all know what it means to need to go to the bathroom to empty our bladder. We recognize how the pressure in our bladder feels and we know how to locate the bathroom. We know what to do when we get there -- meaning how to shut the door, raise or lower the toilet seat, unbuckle our belt and unfasten our pants. We remember how to pull our pants and underwear down, sit down and void, or empty, our bladder. And we understand how to wipe ourselves, flush the toilet and fix our clothing back to how it was before.

We then wash and dry our hands. We open the door and leave the bathroom and return to where we were before. And without hesitation, we resume whatever task or activity we were involved in before we went to the bathroom.

But to a person with dementia, this trip to the bathroom is a complex one. A person with dementia may or may not recognize what the physical clues are or what the urge to void her bladder or empty her bowels mean.

She may no longer recognize what a bathroom is, where it is located, or what she supposed to do in a bathroom. She may have forgotten the purpose of toilet paper or even a toilet. She may not remember how to get her belt undone and her pants unbuttoned and unzipped and down. There are dozens of steps we do without an apparent second thought, because it is memory. And it is a memory of a series of steps you have done countless times.

Memory is everything you know and everything or item or person or the steps you need to be able to exist in the environment around you. And this includes clues from your body about bodily functions like a full bladder, or bathing or chewing and swallowing food.

When we talk about the brain and memory, we are not only talking about actual damage to the brain itself, but also the implied changes in the body's ability to function. This includes changes in personality and behavior, changes in the five senses, changes in the brain's ability to communicate to the body its needs and functions.

In short, what it means for you, the caregiver, when the doctor says, "Your mother has dementia; she's going to lose her memory," is, in reality, a complex statement indicating devastating and drastic changes in your loved one's aging process. In no way does this simple sentence actually prepare you for the difficulties ahead.

The behaviors you may witness from your loved one could include forgetting how to find a bathroom, or accusing you of stealing. It could mean not being able to remember the doctor's appointment, how to dress or operate a car or any of a thousand other behaviors. These changes in memory or behavior are a result of the damage dementia is causing in the brain. And that's the key. Everything your loved one is doing is directly related to damage occurring in her brain. The damage is something you can't see, except in her behavior. For most people, the loss of cellular structure in their brain will only begin to affect the outward physical appearance in the final stages of the disease.

And that is difficult for most caregivers. We expect a person who is sick to look sick. Persons with cancer, AIDS, nausea, the flu or cold or allergies look sick, but people with dementia don't. And because a person with dementia doesn't look physically ill until the very end of the stages, typically not until Stage Six, it is easy for caregivers to forget a disease is causing the behaviors a person exhibits. We have trouble accepting that a dementia process, such as Alzheimer's or Lewy Bodies or FTD, is causing behaviors to appear or change. We have trouble believing the person isn't aware of the behaviors, partly because she doesn't look sick.

For the person with dementia, the diagnosis of dementia may be both devastating and exhausting, mentally and physically. Likewise, the disease is also exhausting to the caregiver. But if you can understand the disease process, you may be able to provide better care at home for a bit longer than you imagined, and not lose yourself in the process. Knowing why a person behaves the way she does doesn't change the behavior, but understanding why she is behaving that way may bring you some measure of relief.

Caregivers really do suffer as a result of providing care for a loved one. Mental and physical health is affected, sometimes to the extreme. Caregivers have some of the highest levels of depression, anxiety and compassion fatigue of any group, but rarely seek assistance from their doctor. Often times, their health is not seen as an issue because the attention is on the person with dementia only. It is imperative that caregivers remember to stop and take care of themselves as well.

Common Reactions to Diagnosis

A diagnosis of any terminal illness, especially dementia, is devastating to the person with dementia and her caregiver. You and your loved one will likely experience significant emotional changes as well following the diagnosis. She may become fearful or paranoid of what is ahead. You may feel grief, disbelief, fear, guilt or even anger. She may take a carefree attitude and appear unfazed by the news, or she may become depressed or saddened.

You may find your reaction is much more emotional. Fear, horror, sorrow, anger, pity and terror are just a few of the adjectives families use to describe their own reaction.

There is also the possibility that you may find yourself in a situation where your loved one can fool a physician unskilled in making a dementia diagnosis. You may leave multiple doctors' appointments with no answers or assistance for the strange behaviors you are witnessing in your loved one. Some caregivers report being told by physicians there are no issues to be concerned about or even that the problems are all in their minds and not the person with dementia! This generally occurs because people are able to use their long-term memories of social skill conversations to appear to be alert and oriented to time, date, self and place.

A person with dementia may ask for your help or she may refuse care or assistance. She may become hostile or suspicious when she forgets that she doesn't remember. Because dementia destroys the brain and because the brain runs the body, in time your loved one will change and undergo the final physical changes of dementia. These changes are typically only seen near the end of the disease. They include a dramatic loss of body weight, a withering of the facial features, a loss of facial affect (emotion), and an inability to be independent in movement. Your loved one may lose her language speech or visual comprehension. She becomes a person totally reliant upon others for survival.

You may find yourself one of the lucky few whose mother quickly and efficiently turns over all her medical and financial care and decisions without hesitation. Or you may discover your mother's dementia has progressed to a point of fear and distrust and paranoia. You may even have to seek legal means to force her to have care under a guardianship.

If your mother has a history of emotional or physical abusive behavior towards you, dementia may intensify this behavior, increasing your stress and guilt. Adult children whose parent had a personality disorder or other major mental illness can find caregiving to be especially difficult. (Try reading the book **Toxic Parents** by Susan Forward and Craig Buck for a new perspective on life.)

These are common scenarios for families and persons facing dementia. Although dementia follows a fairly predictable path, each affected person and family is different. What works for one family may not work for yours. There are no easy solutions.

The decisions you will have to make are going to be difficult. Remember each of us is human, and each of us is unique in our own development, our own aging process and how we approach challenges. Knowing you will need to provide care for your loved one over the coming months or years can be overwhelming.

But by learning what dementia is, you will be better prepared for the challenges ahead. If you and your family can understand what dementia is doing to your loved one's brain and how damage to the brain turns into physical and emotional behaviors during the different stages of the disease, that knowledge will change how you respond to the disease.

I firmly believe if you understand what the disease is doing to her brain, you are better prepared as a caregiver.

In decades of working as a geriatric social worker and then as a gerontologist, I have yet to meet a family who completely understood what a diagnosis of dementia would mean to them and their loved one. It is rare for a physician to explain the dementia process and what the disease will do to the person's brain and how a damaged brain functions.

This is not because the doctor is not competent, but because dementia is a complicated disease and the explanation of the disease process is not the physician's job. Doctors don't have the hours of time needed to explain a complex medical and behavioral disease, nor is teaching a patient about the disease a part of a physician's training or expertise. Unfortunately, this means entire families are woefully unprepared for the emotional and physical changes that will accompany the diagnosis as dementia progresses.

Being told dementia will cause your loved one to have memory problems is just the tip of the iceberg. Dementia is not just a "memory problem." Dementia is a devastating and terminal disease. Yes, unfortunately, it gets worse.

Should a person live to the end of the disease process, she will experience the total loss of her abilities, talents and personality. She will lose all or most of her physical, mental and emotional traits. The disease process of dementia causes the loss of those complex behaviors that make each individual different, each one of us unique.

Caregivers with a better understanding of the cause of the behaviors exhibited by their loved one will automatically become better advocates for their loved one. You will be better prepared to distinguish your loved one's behaviors from your emotions. You will be able to separate and recognize those behaviors as disease driven. You will be ready to successfully face the years ahead.

Granted, knowing about the process of dementia won't change the facts of the disease. But you may be able to change your approach as you face what at first may seem to be a seemingly unending series of uncharacteristic or bizarre behaviors over the next months and years. By the end of this book, you should be able to associate those behaviors with damage occurring in specific lobes of the brain.

Being able to connect your loved one's behavior to the damage in specific areas of the brain probably won't lesson your pain. It should, however, give you a better understanding of why your loved one is behaving the way she is. It will allow you to provide better care at home, and clear oversight when your loved one requires placement in a community.

Remember a person with dementia cannot change what is happening to her. We are the ones with three pound brains, we are the ones who can change our behavior.

Diagnosing Dementia

Recently Dr. Ronald Devere, a board certified neurologist who specializes in dementia, led the team that posted the diagnostic criteria for making a dementia diagnosis. The information is available through the Department of Health and Human Services in Texas and can be downloaded for free. The criteria is designed for a general practitioner to be able to follow the series of tests, including oral, cognitive and laboratory criteria, to make a correct diagnosis of dementia, including specific forms of dementia. The webpage is www.dshs.state.tx.us/ alzheimers and the PDF is entitled ***Clinical Best Practices for Early* Detection, Diagnosis, and Pharmaceutical and Non-Pharmaceutical Treatment of Person's With Alzheimer's Disease.** If you do not have an available computer and printer, contact your Area Agency on Aging and request a copy of the criteria. Share it with your physician and family members or support group and be sure to ask questions about any portion you don't understand.

Five Points To Remember

1. Dementia is now seen as an umbrella term for four dozen (or more) types of brain disease.
2. Memory is everything you and I are able to do.
3. The process of memory is very complex.
4. Being devastated by your loved one's dementia diagnosis is normal.
5. Understanding what dementia is and what it will do to your loved one's brain will make your job as a caregiver easier.

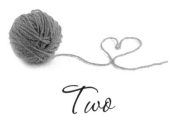

Two

History of Dementia and Alzheimer's Disease

You are not alone in your efforts to provide care for your loved one. Dementia doesn't care about your loved one's education, intelligence, social status, background, career, gender or age. It is a complex and overwhelming group of diseases affecting the brain and hence everything about the person.

Medically speaking, dementia is a general term for a decline in mental ability to a point where it interferes with daily life – the cognitive, social and familial functioning required of all individuals. At least two of the four lobes of the brain must be affected for your loved one to have a dementia diagnosis. Expect that by the end of the disease, all four lobes will be impacted.

A more complete medical description would be that dementia is a term describing different disorders characterized by the development of multiple cognitive impairments, including memory loss, and they are directly related to a general medical condition occurring in the brain.

Some dementias are more common than others (Alzheimer's affects the most people). Some are proven to be genetic (Huntington's or Early Onset Alzheimer's). Others seemingly strike at random (Frontotemporal Dementia). Some are caused by our own behavior (playing a sport that allows you to be repeatedly struck in the head or sniffing paint). And a rare few strike children such as Niemann-Pick's Disease or Huntington's.

It is also not uncommon to find people who have multiple dementias. For example, Lewy Body Dementia and Parkinson's Dementia may appear together or a person with Vascular Dementia may live long enough to develop Alzheimer's as well. This is called dual dementia or Mixed Dementia. That means two separate dementias are attacking that person's brain. There are even recorded cases of persons with three or four distinct dementias.

So to work through what dementia is, who is at the highest risk, how it attacks the brain, what behaviors began to appear or which abilities are lost first – let's just start at the beginning and where we get the words.

Pinel's Word "Demence"

The formal discovery of Alzheimer's disease process is fairly recent. In his book **How We Die**, Dr. Sherwin B. Nuland writes the word dementia comes from a French physician named Philippe Pinel. In 1801, Pinel coined the word "demence" to mean "incapacitation of the mental facilities" as he described an unusual disease process he was witnessing in a patient. The woman, who was in her early 30s, had suffered severe declines in her mental and physical health.

Now before you start to think "Oh no, she was only 34!" remember that life spans were much shorter in the past. In 1801, for example, a person in her 30s was considered old. As medical science advanced, diets improved and clean water became available, our population began to live longer. In 1850, a 40-year-old person was considered old. In 1900, a 50-year-old person was considered old. In 1950, a 60-year-old person was old.

Today, a person turning 65 in the United States or other first-world countries can expect to live an additional 17 years. When you add in the size of the baby boomer population, this makes our aging population the fastest growing demographic group in our country. So don't panic about the age of Pinel's patient. What's important for you to remember is that it was from this woman and her physician that we get the word dementia.

These disease processes we now call dementia have actually been detailed in Western literature for thousands of years. Even the earliest writings of medicine describe behaviors, illnesses and deaths that could only be caused by one of the dementias. Believe it or not, you already know this. Think about kings and emperors who went "mad" or references to people who had "shaky disease." They are easy to find in history and literature. "Shaky disease" would obviously be Parkinson's, while instances of rulers who became paranoid and accused their children of robbing them could be a manifestation of a classic Alzheimer's disease behavior.

Growing up, I heard adults describe an elderly person as "confused" or "senile." As a child, I was told certain elderly people displaying odd behaviors had developed "hardening of the arteries." We now recognize these disease processes as forms of dementia instead. "Hardening of the arteries" is now known as Vascular Dementia and "senility" is Alzheimer's disease. (The terms "senility"and "hardening of the arteries" are no longer used in medicine.)

We now know that over the course of just a few years, a person with dementia may lose her ability to pay attention enough to be able to follow conversations or actions, and she may become apathetic, angry, agitated or even aggressive. These commonly described behaviors occur because the person with dementia is reacting to her brain not functioning as it normally would.

Think about it. She is frustrated, depressed, annoyed, all of the things you and I would be if our brains weren't able to process information as quickly as we were accustomed to.

Imagine for a moment how you would feel if everyone around you began to suddenly insist the year was 2045. At first you might think it was funny. But as they continued to insist the date was decades from what you remember, how would you respond?

Would you become alarmed when your own memories didn't match that year or that decade? Would you become paranoid, frightened or even angry? Would you try to argue the "correct" time? Would you begin to be afraid that something terrible was wrong with you because you didn't remember the lost decades of time? Would you be suspicious of the person who insists the year is 2045?

These would, be and usually, are responses of a person with Alzheimer's. In the beginning, she may laugh off your insistence about the date. Later she may not appear to care at all about the date. But in between those two periods, she undergoes a great deal of fear and frustration, often because her brain can't find the experiences from decades gone by or she can only find bits and pieces of each memory.

As the disease progresses, the person with dementia will lose the ability to use short-term or long-term memory (amnesia), the ability to use or understand language (aphasia); the ability to display appropriate emotion (apathy), the ability to recognize or use common objects or people (agnosia), and the ability to use coordinated muscle movement (apraxia). She will even display an inability to recognize that she has an impairment of cognition (anosognosia). **This means people with dementia aren't pretending they don't remember they have dementia, it means they really don't remember they have dementia.**

"I Have Lost Myself."

Nuland also wrote about Dr. Jean Esquirol, a student of Pinel's. Esquirol treated a female patient in 1838 with similar behaviors to Pinel's patient. Following her death, Esquirol performed an autopsy and documented the damage and changes he saw in the woman's brain.

"Convolutions of the brain are atrophied, separated from one another or flattened, compressed and small, especially in the frontal regions," he wrote. Esquirol's observations were similar to those made years earlier by Pinel, who described areas of his patient's brain as "depressed, atrophied, and almost destroyed, and the empty space filled with serum."

Basically, both physicians determined the women's brains had shrunk dramatically in size and were full of fluid.

Less than 100 years later, on November 4, 1906, a 39-year-old German physician presented his case study of a woman who had displayed unusual behaviors and paranoia in the months and years before her death. At that meeting, for the first time, Dr. Alois Alzheimer spoke about a form of dementia that would, by 1910, bear his name.

He had been on duty on November 25, 1901 when a woman named Auguste Deter was admitted into a psychiatric hospital in Frankfurt, Germany. The woman's family had brought her to the hospital because of her increasingly erratic behavior. During admission, Dr. Alzheimer took detailed notes of her responses to his questions as he attempted to gather her family and medical history.

While his discovery and lecture are well documented, less was known about Dr. Alzheimer's interview with Auguste. The chart on her case had simply been lost. You can now Google the name Auguste D. and find photographs of both her and Dr. Alzheimer. I find the look of late stage dementia to be clearly present in her photo.

The file on Auguste was finally found on December 19, 1995. It was two days after the commemoration of the 80th anniversary of Dr. Alzheimer's death. Eventually his notes were translated and published in the May 24, 1997 edition of **The Lancet.**

The chart has Auguste's admission report and case history. Dr. Alzheimer's notes of his interactions with Auguste are strikingly, painfully familiar. I have included portions of his notes from **The**

Lancet's article. They are chilling in that these original notes could literally be the same for anyone with advanced dementia being interviewed today. (Dr. Alzheimer's notes and questions are in bold; Auguste Deter's answers are in italics).

"November 26, 1901

She sits on the bed with a helpless expression.

What is your name?

Auguste.

Last name?

Auguste.

What is your husband's name?

Auguste, I think.

Your husband?

Ah, my husband.

She looks as if she didn't understand the question. Are you married?

To Auguste.

Mrs. D?

Yes, yes, Auguste D.

How long have you been here? She seems to be trying to remember.

Three weeks.

What is this? I show her a pencil.

A pen.

A purse and key, diary, cigar are identified correctly. At lunch she eats cauliflower and pork. Asked what she is eating, she answers spinach.

When she was chewing meat and was asked what she was doing, she answered potatoes and then horseradish. When objects are shown to her, she does not remember after a short time which objects have been shown. In between she always speaks about twins. When she is asked to write, she holds the book in such a way that one has the impression that she has a loss in the right visual field. Asked to write Auguste D, she tries to write Mrs. and forgets the rest. It is necessary to repeat every word.

Over the next several days, Alzheimer continued to gather information from Auguste. On November 29, 1901 he asked Auguste:

…What year is it?

Eighteen hundred.

Are you ill?

Second month.

What are the names of the patients? She answers quickly and correctly. What month is it now?

The 11ᵗʰ.

What is the name of the 11ᵗʰ month?

The last one, if not the last one.

Which one?

I don't know.

Using her long-term memory, Auguste then correctly identified the colors of snow, the sky and grass. She is able to tell Dr. Alzheimer the correct number of eyes, fingers and legs she has. But then she is lost again.

...If you buy six eggs, at seven dimes each, how much is it?

Differently.

On what street do you live?

I can tell you, I must wait a bit.

What did I ask you?

Well. This is Frankfurt and Main.

On what street do you live?

Waldemarstreet, not, no...

When did you marry?

I don't know at present. The woman lives on the same floor.

Which woman?

The woman where we are living.

The patient calls Mrs. G, Mrs. G, here a step deeper, she lives... I show her a key, a pencil and a book and she names them correctly. What did I show you?

I don't know, I don't know.

It's difficult isn't it?

So anxious, so anxious.

I show her three fingers; how many fingers?

Three.

Are you still anxious?

Yes.

How many fingers did I show you?

Well this is Frankfurt am Main."

Towards the end of the exam, Alzheimer administers a writing test to Auguste. She is not able to complete it and in a statement that perhaps sums up the disease process better than any other she said, ***"I have lost myself."***

When you read the part of the book covering the files and filing cabinet, come back to this section. See if you can determine where Auguste was answering the questions using memory located in her oldest files.

Auguste died on April 8, 1906. Her chart indicates she had developed a decubitus ulcer (also known as a skin breakdown, pressure sore or wound, or a bed sore), she was experiencing high fevers and she had pneumonia in the lower lobes of both her lungs.

Her official cause of death was septicaemia due to decubitus (her blood became septic from the bedsore), various and acute forms of damage in her brain, pneumonia and inflammation of her kidneys.

People with dementia frequently die from developing pneumonia, because the brain can't tell the body how to fight infection. Pneumonia typically develops because they aspirate food particles into their lungs. As the disease reaches its final stages, the brain can no longer tell the mouth and throat musculature how to grab food and swallow it correctly. In the final day or hours of life, it is not uncommon for a bed sore to erupt and the blood quickly becomes septic as a result.

Old Timer's Disease

Alzheimer continued to write about his study of Auguste and the succession of symptoms she displayed before death, including "jealousy, failure of memory, paranoia, loss of reasoning powers, incomprehension, [and] stupor." And when Auguste D died, he performed an autopsy on her brain.

Especially skilled in the newly developed area of tissue-staining techniques, Alzheimer had gained a reputation as the doctor who first identified the changes in cellular structure specific to syphilis, arteriosclerosis and senility. Eventually his techniques and skill with brain tissue would also assist in the study of Huntington's Chorea (another type of dementia).

Today, Alzheimer is best remembered for documenting the changes he saw when he studied slides of Auguste's brain tissue following her death. Using an optical microscope, he determined that between one-fourth and one-third of her brain showed changes in both structure and function. In fact, many cells had disappeared altogether and been replaced with dense bundles of fibrils where the nucleus and the brain cells should have been.

In places where her brain had atrophied and the empty space was filled with cerebrospinal fluid, Alzheimer found bone-like structures made of plaque around the nerve endings. The result of the damage was that Auguste's normal three-pound brain had shrunk to a one-pound brain by the time of her death.

When Alzheimer's mentor Dr. Emil Kraepelin authored his eighth medical textbook in 1910, he included the case study Alzheimer had written about Auguste. Kraepelin titled the chapter "Alzheimer's Disease."

Unfortunately for us, Dr. Alzheimer's name is often mispronounced as "Old Timer's Disease," which helps lead to a myth that as we age, we will all lose our minds and abilities. In reality, most of us will learn new information at the age of 80 at about the same rate we learned when we were 20. The normally aging brain actually becomes more complex as it continues to learn and store information. The dendritic growth of the cells becomes thicker and richer and the "files" of the brain contain more experience and information. Some of the dendrites (roots structures for the cells) in older brains are even several inches long!

As a break and a boost, read **The Mature Mind** and **The Creative Mind** by Dr. Gene Cohen. These are wonderful books and Dr. Cohen discusses the normal aging process of the brain and the extraordinary creativity of older brains.

So the most common dementia is named after the physician Alois Alzheimer, who documented and wrote about the changes he observed in a patient (Auguste Deter's) brain. Likewise, Lewy Body, Huntington's, Pick's Disease, etc., are so named because of the physicians who first documented the disease process.

Dementias are also named from their causation. Vascular Dementia, AIDS Dementia and Chronic Traumatic Encephalopathy (football or boxer's dementia) are named from the event or events causing the dementia. Or dementia may be named because of where it strikes the brain, as is the case in the nine forms of Frontotemporal Dementia (FTD) -- the frontal and temporal lobes are attacked. Dementias may also be named for major features of the disease as in the example of Primary Progressive Aphasia, which is also classified as an FTD.

Ironically, Alzheimer's conclusion at the end of his report became a universal understatement when he wrote, "We are apparently confronted with a distinctive disease process."

⌒

Five Points To Remember

1. Some forms of dementia are genetic and others seemingly strike at random.

2. A person can have more than one dementia at a time.

3. The most common dementia is Alzheimer's disease.

4. Dementias are named for the doctor who documented or discovered them, or for the root cause of the disease, for the area of the brain where the disease originates or for the primary feature of the disease.

5. Dementia in any form is a terminal disease.

Three

Four Forms of Alzheimer's – So Far

Many caregivers first get lost trying to navigate through dementia by not understanding what the word itself means. Knowing dementia is an umbrella term for several dozen diseases impacting the brain is the first step. The next one is knowing each of these dementias may have several forms or sub-sets.

Are you with me so far? What I am saying is that the word "dementia" means we are talking about at least one of 48 types of identified brain diseases, but that within each dementia there can be a further breakdown into different forms or types. This may sound confusing, but you already understand this concept, just in another disease form.

What If It Was Cancer?

In other words, think about the word "dementia" in the same way you do when you hear the word "cancer."

When people hear the doctor give them a diagnosis of cancer, one of the first things they want to know is what specific type of cancer has been identified. They then expect to be told explicitly how that cancer will affect them or their loved one physically and emotionally and what treatments will be recommended for this particular form of cancer.

The questions they ask are almost automatic. What kind of cancer? What stage has the cancer advanced to? How far it will go? Is medication or treatment available? Is it hereditary? Is it terminal?

They also expect their general or family practice physician to direct them to a specialist (an oncologist) who has additional training and expertise in their particular cancer. This specialist confirms or corrects the diagnosis by one or more forms of testing and helps the family prepare a care plan or course of treatment. We certainly wouldn't stand for a physician who casually remarks to a patient: "You have cancer. I'll see you in about six months."

But this is the type of scenario that often plays out for a person diagnosed with dementia. A physician, usually not a geriatric specialist, sees an elderly person after complaints of memory or cognition issues are brought up. The physician then makes a diagnosis of dementia or Alzheimer's by using a basic orientation test (the Mini Mental Status Exam or MMSE) and looking at the patient's birth date. Testing is usually a quick, verbal and is not comprehensive.

After delivering the news of a possible dementia diagnosis, some doctors simply instruct a patient to come back in several months for another checkup. Or they may prescribe medication designed to slow down Alzheimer's. The family may or may not be told the available medications don't work for everyone. Indeed, only about half of the people with Alzheimer's benefit from medication. Others have adverse reactions. There are some people whose specific type of dementia contraindicates the use of dementia medications at all.

But in too many cases, the doctor does not refer the patient to specialist. Families don't get an explanation of the medications. Nor do they get information about dementia and its different forms. Many families I see believe dementia is one disease and Alzheimer's is another. And far too many families may find themselves in a rural or semi-rural area where no other doctors or specialists are available to make a diagnosis.

If this happens, a family must proactively step in and demand a specific dementia type diagnosis so that an appropriate course of action can be put into place. Just like the patient who receives a cancer diagnosis and goes for a second opinion from a specialist, a patient who receives a dementia or Alzheimer's diagnosis from a general practitioner should expect a referral to an experienced neurologist, geriatric psychiatrist or geriatrician. At the very least, try to locate an internist with a geriatric specialty.

Remember to just keep comparing your response of a dementia diagnosis to cancer. If the cancer is in a specific area, you will automatically ask more questions. Do so here. For example, if your doctor told you the illness is breast cancer, you would ask and be told which breast cancer you are facing. If it is bone cancer, you would be told which bone cancer. In other words, cancer has types and subtypes, and the same questions should be expected from the specialist in a dementia diagnosis. If it is Alzheimer's, ask which Alzheimer's. If it is Vascular Dementia, ask which Vascular Dementia.

At present, there is a spinal fluid test that will diagnose Alzheimer's disease, so families don't have to wait for an autopsy to have a diagnosis. There are also new dye scan tests (PET) that highlight proteins and plaque buildup in the brain and identify several forms of dementia with accuracy. Cognitive tests such as the SLUMS or Montreal tests can alert professionals to a potential problem and quickly allow for further testing.

A full diagnosis typically comes only comes after one of these specialists performs a battery of tests that likely will include full cognition testing, blood and laboratory testing, an MRI, and possibly other neuropsychological exams, an EEG, an EKG, PET scans and/or CAT scans. There are more than two dozen specific tests involved in determining which form of dementia a person has. The initial exam by the neurologist should take at least an hour and it normally takes about three visits for the neurologist to make the final diagnosis.

Another reason to expect and demand proper testing is that a variety of common medical events that mimic cognitive difficulties and often look like a dementia are actually treatable with medications. The most common of these is depression, or pseudo-dementia. Others include hormone imbalances, vitamin deficiencies, thyroid changes, low-grade infections or even the lack of socialization.

A 100 percent diagnosis can be confirmed through a spinal tap or brain biopsy or after death when brain tissue is examined through a brain autopsy. And remember the new injectable dye and PET test? This new test makes a definitive diagnosis of the form of dementia and helps the doctor and family prepare a plan of care and treatment. Many times patients find this exam is expensive, more than $4,000 and not covered by insurance.

Like cancer, dementia also has a staging method to follow the progression of the disease, allowing families to track the advancement of the disease and plan accordingly for care needs. The seven stages of dementia (The Reisberg Global Deterioration Scale) and the Dementia Behavioral Assessment Tool (DBAT) are discussed later in this book.

The DBAT can be downloaded for free from www.tamcummings. com and the GDS can be found online.

So Alzheimer's disease is one of the dementias rather than a separate disease and it is the largest group of dementias. Let's start with the most common form of Alzheimer's.

Regular Onset Alzheimer's Disease--DAT

An estimated 52 to 54 percent of persons diagnosed with dementia have regular onset Alzheimer's disease. Its technical or medical name is Dementia of the Alzheimer's Type or DAT. This is the Alzheimer's diagnosed when a person is in her sixties or seventies and begins to show challenges with cognition and memory.

It is the Alzheimer's most frequently referred to in research or the media. And it is the most common form of dementia.

This person will, without any additional medical complications, follow the stages of dementia with what is known as "The Slippery Slope." Meaning this person will move progressively from one stage to the other.

But because most people are not diagnosed until Stage Five of the disease, death usually occurs within five to 10 years of diagnosis. In reality, it is now believed that persons with DAT actually had the disease process begin in their 40s, but the complexity of the brain and its attempts to repair itself delay us from being able to identify the disease earlier. The complexity of the brain allows for the person with dementia to continue to function at a high level and in effect "fool" others around her. (The entire set of stages and corresponding behaviors are covered in the Chapter Twelve.)

Early or Younger Onset Alzheimer's Disease

Another subset of Alzheimer's is: Early or Younger Onset Alzheimer's (EOA or YOA). This dementia strikes from preteen or teen (very rare) up to a person in her fifties. This is the Alzheimer's linked genetically within family groups. Currently an estimated 18 genes have been identified and linked to this form of Alzheimer's. Some families have also been identified as having multiple sets of these genes, indicating earlier and more aggressive onset.

In this type of dementia, the family would most commonly have a history of family members including grandparents, aunts, uncles, cousins, etc., dying in their thirties, forties fifties and early sixties. A book on one such family is **The Thousand Mile Stare** by Gary Reiswig. And although doctors can test for the genes in person's concerned about a family history of dementia, many doctors will refuse to do so. The reason is because even though the genes are identifiable, not every one with the gene will develop Alzheimer's. So it is possible to have the gene, but not have the disease, and as of yet, this is not understood.

Early or Younger Onset Alzheimer's also appears to strike the brain in a different manner than regular onset Alzheimer's. Scans reveal a much different beginning and progression of the disease. Rather than starting in the hippocampus area and sweeping through the temporal lobes and moving forward through the frontal lobes and backwards through the occipital lobes and ending in the parietal lobes, this dementia hits different lobes in the brain almost at the same time. The effect is more like firecrackers, exploding outwards in the parietal and frontal lobes.

A person with this dementia will advance rapidly through the stages, because of the type of dementia and the younger age of the person. The younger someone is when dementia appears, the more aggressive the disease is. The time of disease progression suggested in the stages of dementia would fall more towards the rapid progression, rather than the slower one. For example, if the stage is one to three years, we would anticipate this person will move through the stage in one year, rather than three.

This person is typically diagnosed faster than persons with regular onset Alzheimer's, because the behaviors are viewed as being odd for a young person and there may be a familial link, that is, other family members who also display an early loss of cognitive ability. And remember, the younger a person is when she develops dementia of any kind, the more rapid the progression of the disease.

Because this Early Onset Alzheimer's dementia is so aggressive, death occurs within five years or so of diagnosis or typically before the age of 65.

Down's Syndrome and Alzheimer's Disease

Alzheimer's and Down's Syndrome is another sub-set. It is now accepted that a person with Down's who lives long enough will develop this form. It is thought that the extra copy of chromosome 21 in the brain leads to an increase of amyloid beta protein. DAT is also associated with a higher production of amyloid beta. The effects of the increased amyloid beta are that as it accumulates in the brain it causes the loss of neurons. The effect of both actions, the accumulation and the neuron loss, are critical in Alzheimer's.

Symptoms in people with Down's are usually seen around the age of 40 to 50. Death occurs only a few years later. The early symptoms of confusion, wandering and disorientation are usually not recognized and are therefore not diagnosed. Behavior changes appear as an exaggeration of the person's normal traits, such as increased stubbornness. Or she may become easily agitated or aggressive.

Other features may include forgetting the names of people she should know, changes in sleeping and eating habits, either eating more or less or sleeping more or less than normal. Family members may notice a change in abilities to make decisions, chose clothes or maintain a normal grooming routine. Some persons also develop a hypersensitivity to sounds. Normal white noise like a ceiling fan, the air conditioning coming on, the dog walking across the floor or doorbells may increase agitation.

Social skills tend to be lost earlier than with other forms of Alzheimer's and may even alert the family and the physician to the diagnosis. She may demonstrate difficulty learning new tasks, get lost in her normal routine and begin having problems with hygiene, toileting or dining skills earlier than persons with other forms of dementia.

During Stages Four and Five, communication will greatly reduce and behavioral problems may begin to be a challenge. These changes are usually presented with a faster decline than regular onset Alzheimer's.

As the disease progresses, she will appear to be almost comatose and interact very minimally with her surroundings. She will be a greater risk earlier for choking or swallowing problems.

She is more likely to have epileptic seizures and may develop psychotic behaviors. Previous social skills will be rapidly lost, much sooner than other forms of Alzheimer's. Families are also under greater levels of stress. A lifetime of wondering "Who will care for my child when I die?" is no longer a question, but instead the realization that you will walk this child to the grave.

There is an additional complication of placement in a memory care community. Many of the national communities have rules about being able to only accept persons with a primary diagnosis of dementia. For persons with Down's Syndrome, this form of Alzheimer's is not the primary diagnosis, so additional efforts to secure care may be required by the family.

Late Onset Alzheimer's Disease

The last subset is known as Late Onset Alzheimer's (LOA). This dementia is one seen in persons in their mid to late eighties or nineties. This population has the possibility of almost a one in two chance of developing this dementia. At age 90, the odds are 43 percent.

While the reasons for this increase in dementia are not known with certainty, it is assumed the disease is linked to the great age of this group. After all, while for the first time in history we are witnessing a large population of persons in this age group, most people still won't live to be 85 or 90 or older.

This dementia is a much slower progressing dementia than other forms. The person diagnosed with LOA is more likely to die from old age related causes, rather than dementia itself. However, Stages Six and Seven are very similar to the reaction of the body at the end of life, so the staging tool is still valid for this age group.

Interestingly, the more socially active this person is, the greater chance she will experience or display only early stage or milder symptoms of the disease. This need for socialization is critical in the care of our elderly. Typically most of our socialization comes from family, friends, neighbors, our churches or synagogues, our work, etc.

But a person of great age may have outlived many of her family and friends. She may be physically impaired and unable to attend services with her religious group, and her neighbors may have changed. Keeping an older person socially active is one of the reasons why persons with dementia typically fare better in communities.

Numbers for Alzheimer's in the U.S.

One of every eight Americans age 65 or older (13 percent) has Alzheimer's. The estimated total for Alzheimer's is 5.3 to 5.7 million.

- Nearly half the people ages 85 and older (43 percent) have Alzheimer's disease.

- Almost two-thirds of all Americans living with Alzheimer's are women. This is because women generally live longer than men, not because women are more likely than men to develop dementia.

- Alzheimer's is the fourth-leading cause of death in the U.S. for those who are age 65 or older. Ischaemic heart disease (heart attack), stroke and other cerebrovascular diseases and trachea, bronchus and lung cancers are one, two and three.

- By 2030, the number of people age 65 or older who will develop Alzheimer's is estimated to reach 11 million, a 50 percent increase from the number of people currently diagnosed. By 2050, that number is expected to reach more than 17 million Americans, triple our current number, if medical developments are discovered to prevent or effectively treat the disease. This increase in numbers is because of the size of the baby boomer population, not because people are "catching" dementia.

- Nearly 15 million Americans provide unpaid care for a person with Alzheimer's disease, an estimated $215 billion of care. Family caregivers provide about 80 percent of this care at home.

The Real Dementia Numbers

Now since Alzheimer's only accounts for about 54 percent of all the dementias, the total of the numbers you just read for dementia are also short by about 46 percent. Including the numbers for persons with all forms of dementias would mean the following estimates:

*Currently 10 million Americans have some form or type of dementia.

*By 2030 the total number of persons with dementia of some form will be 19 million Americans.

*By 2050 the total number will be 32 million Americans with some form of dementia.

*Nearly 28 million Americans are currently providing unpaid care for family members, of which the dollar value is approximately $400 billion.

⟜

Five Points To Remember

1. **Thinking of dementia in terms like cancer may help you better plan for your loved one's care.**
2. **While there are about 48 types of dementia, several of these also have different forms or sub-sets.**
3. **Alzheimer's Disease has four subsets: Early or Younger Onset, Regular Onset or Dementia of the Alzheimer's Type, Down's Syndrome Alzheimer's and Late Onset Alzheimer's.**

4. An estimated 5.3 to 5.7 million Americans are thought to have some form of Alzheimer's.

5. If you take into account all the dementias, more than 10 millions Americans have dementia of some form.

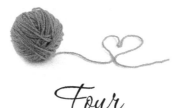

Four

DEMENTIA IN THE BRAIN

More has been learned about Alzheimer's disease in the past 15 years than in the century since its official discovery. The American Psychiatric Association describes Alzheimer's disease as a "multifaceted loss of intellectual abilities, such as memory, judgment, abstract thought, and other higher cortical functions, and changes in personality and behavior."

For most people who develop Alzheimer's, the symptoms typically aren't noticeable to others until the person with the disease reaches her mid-60s. Even then the majority of persons are not diagnosed with Alzheimer's for a few more years or until the disease process advances beyond the middle stages, because the behaviors aren't severe enough to change how a person is safely functioning.

Or it may be that the person refuses her family's attempts to get her to see a physician. Or it may be that you were able to convince her to see a doctor, but she was able to use her social skills so well she could pass initial questioning and the

MMSE. Remember the beginning symptoms of dementia are very subtle and the MMSE was not designed to diagnosis dementia.

In fact, the SLUMS or Montreal Tests can alert a physician to dementia about five years earlier than the MMSE. (Guess which one your insurance company wants used?)

So by the time a person with dementia is finally diagnosed, she may be entering the late stages of the disease and significant damage has already occurred. Most people have approximately four to nine years left before the disease will end their lives. This late diagnosis is why you may read news stories stating most people diagnosed with Alzheimer's will die within five years – it is because the person wasn't diagnosed until late in the disease process.

This late diagnosis of dementia is not only true for persons with Alzheimer's. Unfortunately in most cases, the person with any form of dementia is not diagnosed until the middle or late stages of the disease.

As I said earlier, new research also appears to indicate the disease may cause plaque to begin to build in a person's brain as early as her 40s, although symptoms only begin to show in her 60s. This would indicate the disease is even more complex than previously thought, and that the brain is actually fighting a battle and under assault for several decades before anyone is aware.

This research also underscores the depth and complexity of the human brain – an organ whose estimated 100 billion brain cells perform trillions of activities each nanosecond. The brain uses an identified four dozen or so types of chemicals called neurotransmitters in its function of sending and receiving input from the rest of the body and the surrounding environment.

Some of these neurotransmitters you have heard about. Serotonin, for example, is the main mood-regulating chemical, and the one targeted by anti-depressants. Adrenaline is the neurotransmitter that allows us to react with great strength or speed when we are frightened. It is the one you read about when a woman lifts a car off of her injured child.

In addition to the various cellular structures and chemicals, the brain also requires an internal electrical charge to cause the chemical interactions.

Glucose and the Brain

For most of us, our brains weigh about three pounds. (Men's brains are slightly larger by an ounce or two because males have larger body muscle mass to move.) That translates to between one and three percent of our total body weight. Yet your brain uses 20 to 25 percent of your daily energy supply. Now you know why you feel exhausted after a hard day at work or after you study or concentrate for a long period of time. Your brain is burning up energy!

This tremendous use of energy also helps explain the connection between why a person with dementia and diabetes may experience a more rapid progression of the dementia. The nature of diabetes and the challenges of glucose regulation and exchange in the bloodstream impact the decline from dementia. The brain, damaged by dementia, is unable to draw glucose from the blood supply as it passes through the brain.

Because the brain can't take in its normal energy supply from the blood stream, the effect is a slow starvation of the brain. Altered levels of glucose in the blood stream make this problem even more difficult for the brain of a person with diabetes as it tries to take in energy.

The brain's complexity helps explain why the disease of dementia can take so long to be noticed. It is why a person is able to function at high levels or appear as though she really knows and understands what is happening around her for so many years. This gets complicated here, so let's start with the numbers.

A Million, A Billion and A Trillion

We all hear the numbers million, billion and trillion on a pretty regular basis. These three numbers are repeated during our daily or weekly routines: million, billion, and trillion. So and so is a millionaire, that company sold for a billion dollars, the nation's debt is trillions. But trying to really understand what those numbers mean helps us understand why Mom is able to do a task one moment and not the next – or vice-versa.

Remember, she had 100 billion cells doing trillions of activities per second. Say that again to yourself. She had 100 billion brain cells doing trillions of activities per second. Those are incredible numbers, but hard to grasp in everyday terms.

You can think of the numbers like this. If I wanted to count to a million, and I wanted you to sit with me, we would need to order some food. To count to just one million would take about 34 days. It gets harder as we increase the numbers. To count to a billion would take more than 400 years.

Part of the reason is the sheer volume of that number. The other is it takes longer to say nine billion four hundred million three hundred thousand. You get my point? So to count to a trillion then would be about 200,000 years.

Say it again. My brain has 100 billion brain cells doing trillions of activities per second. This complex mass of brain connections is why a person with dementia can have moments of lucid thought in the midst of advanced dementia. It is because the brain is very intricate and is still trying to find a pathway to send messages even when it is severely damaged.

Even knowing this, for many families the end result of any of the dementias, especially Alzheimer's, can appear to be a set of seemingly bizarre and confusing behaviors. In reality, the specific behaviors that accompany the disease are quite logical given the damage occurring in the brain.

These behaviors supply the clues that allow us to determine which lobes of the brain are being damaged, or attacked, and the stage of the disease – all critical elements that help families to prepare financially and emotionally for the future of their loved one.

Unlike normal aging, dementia is a "use it until it is gone" disease. Then you figure out the next level of a person's skills and start over. Until the next decline and then you start again. People with dementia are going backwards. Developmental theorists determine at what age a baby, then an infant, a toddler, then a child, pre-teen, teenager and young adult develop, emotionally and physically. You can review these stages from Dr. Eric Ericson's Psychosocial Stages of Development. In dementia, people's abilities are going backwards. This scale is referred to as Alzheimer's Retro Genesis (back to the beginning) Scale.

As dementia progresses throughout the brain and as the brain becomes more and more damaged, persons with dementia return to the responses and behaviors of infancy.

The Demented Brain

The body undergoes a slow and gradual aging process and the brain does the same. There are some anticipated changes with age, but for the most part, the brain remains highly functional. Despite slight structural differences, the normally aging brain of a mature person is actually quite powerful and complex.

Normally aging people are not at all the stereotyped befuddled and confused elderly person often portrayed on television. Any changes in brain function that occur with aging are more than likely related to the fact that people are no longer using their brains as they did when they were younger.

The older brain has a dense and rich dendritic growth system. It has more "files," more life experiences. Slight hesitations in responses are related more to slowed reflexive action than to a damaged brain. Think about the Olympics for a moment. Who do we send to these games? We send teenagers and young adults because their reflexes are faster.

In people with Alzheimer's or other dementias, the various organ systems of the body age in a way similar to their peers, up to a certain point. But the major difference between them and their non-Alzheimer's contemporaries is in the brain where the disease causes massive structural changes.

A brain damaged in this way is unable to send or receive signals from that person's organs, is unable to call up memories or language, is not as efficient at fighting infection, and is unable to do all the other things that make us individuals. These changes are so significant that, at the final stage of the disease, the body ceases to be able to live, because the brain can no longer operate the body systems.

Physical Changes in the Brain

Knowing what is happening to a brain that's being attacked by Alzheimer's is critical for any caregiver. It can help you better understand the changes you see in your loved one are actually a result of a physical disease, rather than a conscious or purposeful act on the part of that individual.

A diagnosis of Alzheimer's disease normally means four distinct physiological events are taking place in the brain. These four changes mean every lobe of the brain is eventually affected and the behaviors your loved one exhibits are a direct result of these changes.

The Brain Shrinks

- The sulci, or outer folds of the brain, normally lay tightly folded against each other as the brain is snuggled in the cranium. These are the characteristic wrinkles we see when we look at a photo of the brain. During the dementia process, these folds shrink and shrivel so much that you could place your finger or a pencil between the grooves in a space that didn't exist before the disease.

- At this point, the shrinking brain, no longer tightly contained within the cranium, has a half-inch or more of space between the brain and the skull. Once each cell dies, it is removed from the brain tissue by the normal process of the body. (When cells die in the body, circulation removes them to waste and they are voided out either through the bowel or bladder.) As this shrinkage continues, major areas of the brain begin to die and the structure begins to fill with cerebrospinal fluid where cells once were.

- This shrinkage, or atrophy of the cerebral gyri, causes major damage in the areas of the brain controlling higher function, such as memory, language, learning and judgment.

- If you were studying this view of the brain, the impression would be that of a shriveled pecan. The pecan shell looks normal, but when the shell is opened, the pecan is shriveled and not plump. In the early stages, the person looks normal, even though the brain is undergoing significant changes — and is no longer plump.

The Ventricles Enlarge

- The center part of the brain is destroyed and completely missing in the end. This part of the brain consists mainly of the temporal lobes and the back of the frontal lobes, the two parts of the brain that makes a person unique. Remember if you place your hands over your ears, you have located the temporal lobes, the part of the brain that controls language, hearing, memory and smell. And if you place your hand over your forehead, you have located your frontal lobes.

- The frontal lobes contain a person's memory, speech, personality, cognition, attention, judgment, imagination and rational thought. Normally, these lobes have a small bit of cerebrospinal fluid in them in an area called the ventricles. This part of the brain resembles the wings of a butterfly.

- By the end stages of Alzheimer's, large portions of these parts of the brain will be gone and replaced with cerebrospinal fluid. The ventricle area will have enlarged to several times its original size. Damage to these lobes, especially the frontal lobes, is what most impacts a person's personality traits and memory.

Neurofibrillary Tangles

- The nucleus in individual brain cells comes apart. The tau proteins that support the structure of the dendrites (roots of the cells) tangle and the cell dies. In normal functioning brains, the tau proteins are essential to a person's central nervous system.

- In an Alzheimer's patient, tau proteins incorrectly gather and clump within the cell's dendrites. They literally fold the wrong way and damage the cell. No longer neat and functional, the cell's nucleus is destroyed and replaced with dense bundles of fibrils, neurofibrillary tangles and a buildup of protein clumps.

- The once-neat nucleus is starving and dying and the orderly cellular structure is clumped and tangled. The cell is unable to function normally or process information. These cellular structures, ordinarily laid out in neat tracks (like railroad tracks), are now significantly damaged.

- The cells' dendrites reach out towards each other (like fingers or roots), send and receive electrical impulses carrying neurotransmitters, the chemicals present in your brain responsible for function. Adrenaline, serotonin, glutamate, norepinephrine and acetylcholine are just a few of these chemicals you may have heard about. Imagine these cells are the roots of a plant reaching for each other. The "roots" are separated by a space, called a synapse.

- The body's electrical system fires the neurotransmitter. This electric charge causes the neurotransmitter to jump across the synapse. When this happens with a hundred million or billion cells responding, you get a thought or a movement, that is, the brain functions.

- But in dementia, the cells are being destroyed, one by one. In the beginning, a few damaged or dead cells don't have an apparent impact. In time, as more and more cells are lost, the damage becomes apparent, eventually even to outsiders. The brain can no longer find healthy pathways; the memories or files are damaged and then gone. Your loved one can't function. (But the very complexity of the brain means that sometimes, even in very late stages, the brain will suddenly find a pathway to a working group of cells and for possibly one last time, she will know you.)

Plaque Builds Up

- Plaque accumulates in the brain, in the areas between brain cells. During the course of Alzheimer's, there is a build-up of a protein around the nerve endings in the brain, which forms into plaque. This protein normally breaks apart and reforms without any problem, but in dementia, when it breaks down it fails to reform correctly and becomes instead a hard bone like structure. This is not the same as plaque you may hear about that is associated with the arteries. That type of plaque is a soft and pulpy plaque caused by a buildup of blood cells.

- Brain tissue has a consistency similar to medium tofu, which is very soft, yet firm in texture. The type of plaque associated with Alzheimer's is not soft and pulpy; instead, its consistency is more similar to sand or grit.

- This plaque clumps are often found throughout the brain, further impairing the cellular structures' ability to communicate and function.

- As mentioned earlier, recent research indicates this buildup of plaque may actually begin in a patient's 40s with symptoms not showing until that person reaches her 60s.

As you can see, the overall damage to the brain during the course of the disease is extraordinary and the result is devastating to an individual. By the end of the disease process, a healthy adult brain that weighed three pounds and had 100 billion brain cells – a brain that was normal and allowed your loved one to be the person she was – will only weigh about one pound.

So as you read the last sentence again – the three pound brain now weighs only one pound – you should begin to be able to see that everything your loved one is doing, she is doing because of severe damage in her brain.

Her brain's cells will collapse, disintegrate or become a mass of tangles. Fluid will replace entire areas or sections of the lobes, and clumps of plaque composed of degenerated portions of axons will cluster around cores of beta-amyloid at the nerve endings. Plaque will grow. The remaining 30 billion or so brain cells will be heavily damaged and have great difficulty sustaining life.

How the Brain and Body Connect

As we move forward, remember the brain controls all of your body's organs and systems. The systems and organs do not operate independently of one another. The brain controls everything in the body. This includes blood circulation, breathing, swallowing, and kidney function, respiration and infection control, language, hearing, vision, etc. Eventually, her affected and impaired brain becomes more and more damaged by the disease, her body systems, behaviors and who she is will also be affected.

The impact of the disease can be seen specifically as the disease affects the different lobes of the brain. Remember each lobe is responsible for particular functions, abilities or memories. As lobes are damaged and destroyed, the person you know slips away. As memories dissolve, the person may experience personality changes and, at the same time, her body will slowly cease to work properly.

The brain not only controls how organs physically work, it causes our eyes to be able to move in a certain direction or our mouth to make chewing motions. It also translates incoming signals to allows us to form perceptions of our surroundings. In other words, the brain interprets what the eyes see, the mouth tastes, the ears hear, the nose smells and the skin feels.

So it is the brain allowing us to associate a shape with a specific item (i.e., fork vs. spoon), a taste with something pleasant or sour (i.e., cookie vs. lemon), and so on. With dementia, it's not that the organs lose their ability to physically function in their designed capacity, it is that the brain is losing its ability to interpret signals from the organs. The brain can't send or receive the correct message from the different systems. This affects a person's ability to correctly recognize and interpret objects, sounds, tastes, pain, smells or temperature.

As your mother ages with dementia, she may have difficulty identifying who you are. She may refer to you as a sister or another daughter or as her mom or aunt or cousin or grandmother.

In the beginning, she may just be calling you by the wrong name, something we all do on occasion. Later on, she knows who you are, but she is using the wrong family name out of her memory file of family names. As the disease progresses, and she continues to confuse you with someone else, the confusion is not because she needs new glasses.

Her eye as an organ is functioning the same. But her occipital lobe, the part of the brain that translates what the eye is seeing, is not functioning correctly. The right side of her temporal lobe, which also translates and holds visual memories of pictures and faces, is damaged. And her frontal lobes, containing your memories, are now compromised and also damaged.

Likewise her infection system, normally alerted by the brain to increase white blood cells to fight off infection, no longer receives those signals from the brain. She may complain of being cold. Or not complain, but hold herself as though she is cold.

Again, her brain, specifically her parietal lobe, is damaged. Her body is colder, but her brain can no longer regulate the temperature or tell her how to put on a sweater, turn up the heater, etc. And this sensation of cold occurs year round, not just in the winter.

Her brain may or may not recognize the smell of burning objects or fire. She may not be aware the soup on the stove has scorched or the pot is on fire or that the house burning. Dementia may not allow her to find her way out of a burning house or recognize water too hot to touch.

This happens over and over again, with all the systems in the body. As the brain suffers more and more damage, the body and its senses and organs, work less and less efficiently or not at all.

As you begin to put the pieces of the puzzle together, you see how, in addition to controlling the body's function, the brain also controls all aspects of memory. Many families suspect Alzheimer's and first reach out for a diagnosis when memory losses can no longer be ignored. Again this may be because family members don't live nearby, it may be because mom refuses to see a doctor, or it may be because the doctor simply doesn't address the issue. All of these scenarios happen routinely.

Five Points To Remember

1. **A normal adult brain weighs about three pounds and has 100 billion cells.**

2. **As tau proteins begin to fail in function and become scrambled, the dendrites (or cell roots) where the tau proteins exist become a tangled mass. This is called the neurofibrillary tangle. This causes the cell to be unable to communicate with other cells or draw in nutrition from the blain blood supply. The cell then shrivels and dies. Once the cell dies, it is removed from the brain as waste.**

3. The accumulation of plaque in the brain greatly contributes to the progression of the disease.

4. The brain replaces dead cells with cerebrospinal fluid.

5. The brain shrinks to one pound during the full course of dementia.

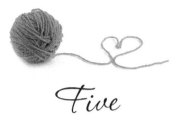

Five

The Filing Cabinet

Remember I've already told you dementia takes a huge structural toll on the brain. For many persons this "toll" is two pounds or so of the original three pounds brain tissue lost as dementia kills the brain cells and the body removes them as part of waste. As we work through what dementia is, sometimes it helps to think of the brain as a set of filing cabinets.

Each of the drawers of the cabinets is full of files. The files in each drawer represent memories. Decades of memories, files of persons or events, files of early childhood, teenage years, young adulthood, parenthood, etc. Every part of a person's life is in a file.

As the disease progresses, the files are corrupted. Typically, the destruction is backwards in time, especially with Alzheimer's. That's why it is no longer this year or this decade, but last year or last decade. The damage in the files is bit-by-bit, piece-by-piece. In the beginning, the disease is very slow. Pieces of information, steps to tasks, names, coordinated moment, gradually these are lost. First a word here or there is lost, then a sentence, a paragraph, a story and finally the file itself is gone. Eventually the brain's memories (files) are empty.

This slow and subtle loss can make it appear as though the person really understands what's happening around her. That she is pretending not to understand or remember. But it is really the brain trying to find information that is forever lost or located in a part of the brain that the cellular structure can no longer reach. It is trapped in a bit of healthy tissue surrounded by holes or badly damaged tissue.

As time goes on and the disease continues, some files are lost completely, while others suffer severe damage. I often hear families complain about how their mother is being "stubborn" or "refuses to do therapy" or some other task. We now know that she is not refusing to participate in therapy or being stubborn or trying to make your life harder, she has damage in her files. People with Alzheimer's simply cannot take advantage of the memories in their files to help with their everyday activities, because the files are damaged or gone.

This means she is not just being stubborn, although it may certainly appear that way. Instead it means everything she does, from recognizing her children to feeding or dressing or cleaning herself, to behaving in a socially acceptable way is happening the way it is, because her files are damaged.

Think about the sudden need to go to the bathroom. Again you and I get up and go without a second thought. We finish and return to the previous task. But for a person with dementia, the corruption of the files by dementia means that memories second nature to a healthy adult will have vanished, because of destroyed brain cells. The bathroom is only one example of what makes up each of our day. The same challenges faced in the bathroom eventually happen in all of our daily activities.

Think about a bath, getting dressed, or cooking a meal. Taking a bath is more than four-dozen steps, starting with remembering you need to take a bath, knowing where the bathroom is, knowing how to undress. It is getting water to turn on or off, be the right temperature. Bathing is knowing what to do, how to do it, knowing you need to rinse the soap off and dry. And then she must know how to dress in clean clothes. The brain and her memories are very complex stuff.

Getting dressed means removing soiled or dirty clothing and replacing those items with fresh clean and appropriate clothing. Making the process more complex are shoes that tie versus slip-ons, or belts, buttons, zippers, and bras. Think about the last one for a second. Bras are pretty complex to get on and off and for the ladies, usually about 10 steps. And there are dozens more for each level or phase of dressing or undressing.

Cooking means remembering how to prepare food to eat and how to remember to prepare safe foods. It means dealing with heat and fire and unspoiled food and pots, pans, seasonings, etc. And it means remembering to turn the stove on and then off after the task is complete.

Memory for persons with dementia also tends to slip away in a reverse chronological manner. We begin storing memories from the time of our birth and we build on those memories throughout life. We learn to hold our heads up, hold our body erect, we lean on our hands and knees and rock, we start pulling up and try to balance, we take a few steps and fall, over and over again. Then suddenly it seems we are walking and running and moving in a coordinated and safe manner. No more bumps on the head, no more bruises on the knees.

The reality is walking is files and files of memory learned over months of time. The files are stored in some very specific brain areas (motor and pre-motor cortex) but also some component of balance and walking and steps and procedures to movement is in different areas or lobes. Alzheimer's disease, and all other dementias, changes all of this, robbing an adult of movement, memories and abilities in the reverse order of how each skill was learned.

This means the most recently stored memories are often the first to go missing. A man in the middle stages of

Alzheimer's disease may be able to describe in detail the first car he bought 50 years ago, but may not remember where he lived after retiring. A woman who can describe her first date in high school may not recognize her grown daughter.

You may already realize your loved one can talk longer about events from the past. That's because these memories, these files, are more deeply embedded. The files are bigger, there's more material there to draw on. There are more of these files stored in the brain and many of them may have been in place since early childhood.

Think about what is in these early files. They include family, social skills, ADLs, language, singing, cursing, movement, etc. First we learn our parents and family, brothers, sisters, grandparents, cousins, aunts and uncles. We learn social skills like "please" and "thank you." We learn an entire conversation known as the social conversation. It starts with "Hi, how are you?" And immediately follows with "Fine, how are you?" This memory is so ingrained in your files, your brain, you don't even think about what the conversation even means. It's automatic.

You learned to dress and color and eat with fingers, a spoon, a fork and finally a fork and knife. You learned to hold a glass and drink without spilling. You learned to bathe.

But now the disease is progressing and everything is going backwards. In time, your loved one will start looking for home, but it is not the home you know. It is the home with Momma and Daddy. Understand?

Use these old files to enjoy time together and help your loved one's world make sense one more time. Respond to the emotion, not the thing said. If she asks or talks about wanting to go home, respond to the emotion of the memory and ask about her home. Ask what her home looked like, smelled like, ask was her mom a good cook? Talk about the ones she loved. You might just find a wonderful memory left in there that's not been heard before.

Martha's Story

Martha was a wonderfully pleasant lady living in Washington, D.C. She was 81-years-old. Her daughter's name was Judi. Judi was 53 and prematurely gray. A loving and kind daughter, Judi visited her mother every day in the dementia community where Martha lived. But the visits were unsettling for Martha. After each visit, Judi was upset, Martha was upset, and the other residents were upset. After meeting with the daughter I went to see Martha.

We exchanged social pleasantries, those "Hi, how are you?" conversations and Martha was fine. Eventually I begin to ask her about her life. Then I asked her if we were a country at war.

"Well of course we're at war," she replied.

"Who are we at war with?"

Giving my question careful thought she replied, "Well, I can't remember his name, but he's got a funny little mustache."

I continued, "Who is our president right now?"

Without hesitating and speaking with what appeared to be great pity for me that I would need to ask her such a question she answered "Why FDR of course."

"What year are we in?"

"Why it's 1944."

To fully comprehend this story, you have to understand what Alzheimer's was doing to Martha's brain and her filing cabinet.

In 1941, Martha moved to D.C. from her small hometown in the mid-west to work at "the War Department." (The Pentagon was called the War Department in WWII). She was one of the millions of women who left their homes and families and relocated to support the war effort. In 1944, Martha was a 24-year-old secretary to an Army general. She didn't meet her husband until 1950 and didn't marry until 1951. Her daughter was born in 1952. Have you solved the mystery?

Because Martha's files are being destroyed in a backward fashion, her current beliefs about time and her orientation have changed. Her reality was not the year 2005 and a war in Iraq, but 1944 and a war with Germany, Japan and Italy.

Every day, her daughter came to see her, always bringing her some chocolate candy. Every day the daughter called Martha "Momma." And every day the daughter said, "I'm your daughter," when her mother would thank her for the candy and then ask who she was. Were you able to solve the mystery?

If Martha thinks is 1944 and she is a single, 24-year-old woman, then how could this "old" woman be her daughter? Martha doesn't remember the year and doesn't understand she is 81 and not 24. In Martha's memories, she can't have a daughter because she didn't remember having a daughter. She didn't recall her husband or her marriage of 48 years because those files were gone, erased by the disease. In her mind, if she doesn't have a husband, she can't be married. If she isn't married, how could she have a daughter?

We solved Martha's daily dilemma by having the daughter continue the visits, but not focus on her role as daughter. Instead she would introduce herself by her name "Judi" and her mother would relax and enjoy the candy as they chatted. Judi became that "nice lady who brings me chocolate," rather than that "strange old woman who calls me 'momma.'" This interaction continued to Martha's death.

In short, what it really means when the doctor says, "Your mother has dementia; she's going to lose her memory," is you can anticipate drastic changes in your loved one's aging process in every aspect of life. The person you love is struggling every day during this disease process to make sense of a world becoming more and more confusing. Hers is a world no longer making sense. Files are lost or the connections between the files are destroyed.

She is doing her best to understand stimuli that no longer have meaning as the disease continues its attack. And some of you have to be comfortable with no longer being the son or daughter or spouse, but instead find peace with becoming that "nice lady who brings me chocolate."

No Going Back

Damage to the brain by Alzheimer's is continuous and aggressive. In the beginning of the disease process, the effects are not as readily seen. They are just not noticeable. Remember the brain starts with 100 billion cells. Even when a few million become damaged, the brain is still able to function by rerouting signals through undamaged pathways for signals to get through.

A thought can still be completed, a sentence can still makes sense, and movement can be completed successfully. When you see your mom misspeak or unable to complete a thought and then, just a few moments later, she makes perfect sense, you are witnessing the brain finding an undamaged pathway.

As the brain suffers devastating cumulative damage during the course of the disease and the brain's ability to interpret and react to the signals and messages becomes more impaired, the impact on the body system's functions are more dramatic. Changes may appear to occur more rapidly towards the end of the disease process because of the cumulative effect of the disease.

Losing a few hundred thousand or even one million brain cells in the beginning doesn't have too much effect because there are so many healthy brain cells still functioning. Toward the final stages of the disease, the changes are detectable in every movement, every facial feature and every component of daily life.

When a specific ability fails because the part of the brain that controlled it is damaged, that ability cannot be regained or relearned. Unlike some other diseases, Alzheimer's does not go into remission. No amount of physical therapy, cueing or coaching or yelling will help. Sadly, this is not a "use it or lose it" scenario.

Instead, this is a "once it is lost, it is gone" scenario. Think of it this way: The brain is the hard drive (the computer's version of the filing cabinet), a sort of the central processor.

All of a person's abilities, personality traits and memories are files stored one-by-one on that hard drive. As the disease progresses, file parts are deleted or erased – a word, a sentence, a phrase, a paragraph – until an entire file is destroyed. Once a file is erased, it is gone. Nothing can be done to recover it. But until that time, the person needs to stay active, socially involved and safe.

Five Points To Remember

1. The brain and its memories are like a filing cabinet and its files.
2. Your loved one's memories started building into "files" from the moment of birth.
3. The files/memories are being removed in an almost backwards fashion.
4. People with dementia can't pretend not to remember something.
5. The oldest files, those from early life, last the longest.

Six

The Four Lobes of the Brain

In most cases, dementia involves an atrophying and damage in the brain either in all four lobes or in a few specific lobes. The type of dementia diagnosed also determines the kind and frequency of damage being done to the brain and the aggressiveness of the disease as it relates to an individual's decline.

Because the brain's functions and structures are far from being completely understood, the disease is even more complex. We are only just beginning to unravel the ways these areas and structures interact with each other. For our purpose, which is to assist families with little or no neurological training understand this disease, we will work with the basics. So let's start at the top.

The brain is divided into many sections, but these various parts fall into four distinct lobes. Each of these lobes is identified as being responsible for certain behaviors, or abilities, that our memories or our bodies are able to do. These four are the frontal lobe, the temporal lobe, the occipital lobe and the parietal lobe.

Each lobe has a left and right side, or hemisphere. During the course of the disease, Alzheimer's will move into and systematically destroy each lobe. As a lobe is destroyed, changes in behaviors specific to that lobe will be evident. Knowing the function of each lobe is critical to understanding the disease process.

As dementia progresses through the brain, it literally destroys the brain by killing individual cells. As the body recognizes these dead cells, it removes them from the body system as waste. The body then replaces the empty space left after the removing of these dead cells with cerebrospinal fluid. In time the damage can be so devastating that a person's brain shrinks from its normal three pounds to only one pound at death. Any dementia is considered to be a terminal disease.

Remember that not every person with dementia will live to the end stage of the disease. Some estimates are that about half of the people diagnosed with dementia will die of other causes before the final stage. In other words, death most likely will result from a cardio or vascular event (heart attack or stroke), the same as most non-dementia people.

If you are secretly hoping for your loved one's death or you have thought to yourself "I hope Mom can go soon," don't beat yourself up. Those thoughts don't make you a bad person, they just make you human.

Stage Seven of dementia means the person is bed bound, incontinent of bladder and bowel, can't speak or recognize others, and is totally reliant upon others for care. I have yet to meet a family that wishes for Stage Seven of dementia for their loved one.

The Hippocampus

Let's talk about how and where Alzheimer's begins for most people.

For you to learn new information, to make a new memory, your hippocampus must be functioning. Located between your ears (roughly), this little structure is the key for making and storing new information. (Its Greek name means sea horse, because of its curled structure.)

When the brain is filtering stimuli around you, the hippocampus is very active. Whether it is a coming birthday for a friend, a doctor's appointment next week, the car in the lane beside you on the road, trust me, your hippocampus is alert and functioning and scanning and recording stimuli.

Ultimately, this structure determines whether information remains short term ("Watch out for the cop!") or long term ("You're going to be a grandmother!"). Its function determines whether or not information is retained in the brain.

Alzheimer's disease starts in the cellular structures below and around the hippocampus. In time, the disease moves into the hippocampus. You witnessed this process and didn't even realize it was happening, because the disease moves slowly in most people.

In the beginning, your loved one repeats questions and you repeat answers because you think her hippocampus is working properly. She asks, you answer, she nods her head and you think she gets the information and stores it.

A simple thing like you telling her the doctor's appointment is next Tuesday at 3 p.m. can drive you mad and make her equally frustrated. She asks about the appointment, you answer her, she nods and you assume she retained the information. And then she asks again, and again and again. Her brain is already damaged, but she doesn't recognize it and she doesn't look sick, so you don't recognize it either.

In reality, once dementia begins to attack the brain, her hippocampus is damaged and eventually can no longer process information. She looks like she understands what you said, but she didn't. Eventually you may get tired of answering the same question over and over and yell at her. Remember people with dementia don't look sick until the disease is almost at the end.

In other words, she doesn't look like her hippocampus is sick because you can't see her hippocampus. Physically she doesn't appear I'll and so much of the brain is still functioning.

But once the repetition of questions begins, the Alzheimer's process is well on its way.

As time passes, because she won't be able to form any new memory, she will begin to use old memory. The stuff in her files still works. You become her mother or grandmother or sister, because those files she can still use. The new grandchild becomes you or another baby she has a file on.

Depending upon the type of dementia someone suffers from, the order in which the lobes are destroyed will vary slightly. In Alzheimer's, the disease starts in the hippocampus, at a point in the front of the temporal lobes and at the rear of the frontal lobes.

It then progresses into the temporal lobes, forward through the frontal lobes and backward through the rest of the temporal lobes before moving into the occipital lobes. At this time it is also moving to the inner top section (cortical) of the brain. Finally the disease will complete a circular route in the brain, ending in the parietal lobe and affecting and destroying all the lobes.

The Temporal Lobes

These lobes are located behind your ears. If you put your hands up around your ears, you are covering the area where you'd find your temporal lobes. These lobes control hearing, language, memory and smell. The left one controls formal language, which is the way you and I speak with each other in general or during social conversations. The right lobe controls a person's ability to recall songs, to curse and to respond with an automatic "yes" or "no" to questions. This is an area where stored information that's deeply ingrained is kept.

In most people with Alzheimer's, the left lobe will suffer greater damage first, before the right temporal lobe. What this means is when the brain cannot use the left lobe to find the correct and appropriate words to respond to a situation, it will resort to pulling out stored information from the right lobe.

That's why a friendly and helpful "Let's change your shirt," can evoke a shocking barrage of curse words your mom would have never even uttered aloud when her brain allowed her to respond with left temporal lobe's socially appropriate behavior.

Mom's new use of cursing vocabulary is especially difficult for families who may be embarrassed, ashamed or simply shocked. Some may be worried this new cursing behavior means she will "go to hell" or that she is damning her soul.

The reality is once you begin to hear curse words being used that were never used in the past, you have an indication the disease has significantly damaged the left temporal lobe. The brain is using stored information from the right lobe to respond to a situation and express (however inappropriately) your mom wants to be left alone or doesn't feel well or is simply having a bad day. "I don't feel good," or "Leave me alone," or "I'm scared," or "I'm having a bad day," may be words and sentences her damaged brain can no longer make. Instead cursing words are used to communicate.

You may be further confused when Mom, who just cursed at you, hears the church service happening on TV or in her community and suddenly sings all the words to the songs. This does not mean she must be able to speak and she is just cursing at you to be mean. The reality is the words to the song are stored information in the right temporal lobe and they can still be recalled.

The same understanding must be extended to any "yes" and "no" answers you receive. "Yes" and "no" are automatic responses learned at a very early age and also stored in the right temporal lobe. Because of the progression of dementia, you cannot rely on them to be correct.

For example, if Mom falls down and hits her arm, you would assume she hurt herself. If you ask, "Does your arm hurt?" and she responds "no," be aware the "no" only has a 50-50 chance of being correct. Her brain is simply responding with a stored language skill that still works and she doesn't truly understand your question.

The Frontal Lobes

The frontal lobes are the lobes behind your forehead. If you were to hold your forehead as though you had a headache, you are covering your frontal lobes. These lobes are what make you an individual. They contain your personality, memory, cognitive thought, executive function, judgment, impulse control, rational thought and speech. They hold family, education and other experiences that shape each of us differently.

The frontal lobes functioning properly keep you from reacting with your true feelings. You may hate a friend's haircut, or you may think that yes, that dress does make her look fat. But because your frontal lobes are working, you may think it, but you would never say it aloud. At least, not to your friend's face.

Dementia damages the frontal lobes and takes away impulse control. The result is language you never expected to hear, rude comments that may embarrass you, names your mother calls caregivers you never heard her use before. This is dementia, not your loved one.

Early in the disease process, you noticed Mom was having trouble with personal finances, struggling to find the right word or repeating the same questions over and over. As the frontal lobe deteriorates, the individual will be unable to recover memories, which are lost in reverse order. This is why a woman will be able to talk about old boyfriends from 50 years earlier, but may not remember her husband or children.

If you are a movie buff, this is the lobe removed from Jack Nicholson's character in "One Flew Over The Cuckoo's Nest." The loss of this lobe reduced the character Mac to someone in need of constant care and no interest in his surroundings.

Inhibition control is also in the frontal lobes. The loss of inhibition can mean everything from aggressive behavior to sexual behavior to any other socially inappropriate behavior. Just hold this thought: everything a person with dementia is doing is a direct result of the damage occurring in her brain. Personality changes, odd fixations of persons or objects, outbursts of behavior, loss of the things that made your loved one unique, these are all happening because of the dementia process.

Everything from swearing, to poor social skills, to inappropriate behavior, to an inability to walk, talk, eat, or dress and clean oneself, are all a result of the disease. It is the dementia.

The Occipital Lobes

The occipital lobes are the lobes located at the lower part of the back of your skull and cradled in the curvature above your neck. These lobes translate what the eyes see and are responsible for vision and depth perception. They also allow you to determine distance from an object.

Working with memories stored in your frontal lobes and temporal lobes, the occipital lobes allow a person to do such things as recognize faces, distinguish one kind of chair from another and translate an environment.

A person's environment is the space she occupies at any given time, whether it is a room in a home, the waiting room at the doctor's office, the long hallway in a community, the tub in a bathroom, the parking lot or the backyard. Although she can physically see these places, her occipital lobe is unable to translate what her eyes are seeing into something that makes sense.

Other signs these lobes are being destroyed include an inability to distinguish day from night, so you might get inquiries about missing lunch at 2 a.m. You loved one also will not be able to separate danger from safety.

For example, she may perceive a shiny, waxed floor as dangerous wet floor and be reluctant to step on it. She may bump into objects or people or walls, she may reach for a glass of water and miss it.

You will know the disease has moved into the occipital lobes when your mom no longer recognizes you, your siblings or her husband, if he is still alive. Remember, her eyes see you but her brain is damaged and your files may be gone. This damage is keeping her from recognizing the person in front of her is someone meaningful and important.

New glasses won't help her at this stage of the disease. Remember it is not her eyes, it is her brain.

The Parietal Lobes

The parietal lobes are located at the top of your head (think of where a Jewish man would place his kippa, or hat). They control and interpret tactile sensation, body temperature and regulation, and pain perception. As these lobes becomes damaged, the person may or may not be able to feel pain, recognize whether the surrounding temperature is hot or cold, or be aware she is being pinched by her waistband.

As you reread the preceding paragraph, you should be starting to realize why your mother is always cold. Or why she doesn't complain about her arthritis anymore. You may begin to understand how a person with dementia craves or only enjoys sweet foods, falls down hard on the floor and doesn't appear fazed, or still enjoys holding your hand.

The severe damage in the parietal lobes means we have to be very careful and watchful of our loved ones. Because her brain is very damaged, we are responsible for keeping her safe and comfortable.

Once the disease has advanced into the parietal lobes, families must be especially alert to their loved one's condition.

⁓

Meg's Story

Recently I was in a memory community where I witnessed a woman stand and turn to move away from the lunch table. Her caregiver noticed the lady went immediately to her room and laid down, an unusual afternoon event for her. Normally Meg would immediately go to the activity area for the after lunch events.

When the nurse arrived, she asked Meg if she felt ill or was in pain. Each time, the woman responded with a "No." When the nurse noticed Meg was lying on her right side instead of her back, she performed a gentle range of motion exam.

Only after the nurse bent the left leg at the knee and began to lift the leg did Meg respond with a very soft "Oh" comment. An x-ray showed a fracture below the ball of the hip joint. For a woman whose parietal lobe was severely damaged, Meg's response to pain was not unusual.

⁓

Five Points To Remember

1. Alzheimer's damages the hippocampus, stopping new memory from being formed. It doesn't matter how many times you repeat information, she cannot learn.

2. The temporal lobes control hearing, language, smell and memory.

3. The frontal lobes control imagination, personality, judgment, rational thought, impulses, speech and memory.

4. The occipital lobes control depth perception and visual acuity.

5. The parietal lobes control taste, touch, temperature and pain.

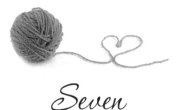

Seven

DEMENTIA, DELIRIUM AND DEPRESSION

Dementia is a slow progressing disease. When you think about your loved one, you should be seeing a decline in abilities that has occurred over a period of several years or months. If you only see your loved one over holidays, then you can almost count backwards from Thanksgiving events and see a steady loss of ability.

Delirium on the other hand, causes a rapid decline in abilities, or the sudden onset of lethargic (slow, sleepy) behavior, or aggressive (agitated, verbal or physical) behavior. It is considered an acute brain dysfunction. The key is your loved one begins behaving much differently than she was only a few hours or days before. Just remember this, dementia is slow, but delirium is rapid and deadly.

Frequently, the cause of delirium is some form of infection. The most common infection in a person with dementia is a Urinary Tract Infection (UTI). Delirium is considered a life-threatening condition for persons with dementia because their systems can be rapidly overwhelmed by the infection. Oftentimes, the changes will take place in a matter of hours.

Think about delirium like this, a UTI won't kill you or me, but it can cause death in a person with dementia. If you notice your loved one behaving differently, look for any causes and call 911 or your mom's doctor.

Physicians recognize the danger of delirium and will respond immediately to your concerns. When you notice sudden changes in behavior, review the delirium mnemonic and match each letter to the sudden change in your loved one. A mnemonic (new-mon-ic) is a way of using an unusual saying or phrase or word to review symptoms of an illness.

DELIRIUM Mnemonic

D (Drugs) Has your loved one had any medication changes or received any new medications, including over the counter drugs?

E (Eyes, ears and other sensory deficits) Has anything happened to change the way your loved one is seeing or hearing in her environment? Or does she have an infection in either her ears or eyes?

L (Low oxygen) Does she have any condition affecting her intake of oxygen? These can include heart attack, stroke, and pulmonary embolism.

I (Infection) Remember UTIs are the most common infection, but also remember colds, flu, etc.

R (Retention of urine or stool or Restraints) Again look for UTI or constipation as a cause for suddenly different behavior. Restraints, either chemical (meaning medications) or physical restraints can cause a person to have behavior changes.

I (Ictal) Has there been a change in glucose, thyroid or lytes levels?

U (Underhydration or Undernutrition) Remember to check for dehydration in an older person; press firmly with your thumb between her eyebrows. When you remove your thumb if you can see the whitish outline of your thumb, then she is dehydrated.

M (Metabolic) This could be caused by a post-operative state or sodium abnormalities.

S (Subdural hematoma or Sleep deprivation) She may have a brain bleed from a fall or ruptured blood vessel or she may be exhausted.

Knowing to watch for and insist your loved one be thoroughly checked when you see a change in behavior is critical as you move forward in caregiving. Treat the symptoms, but seek the cause is a good rule of thumb. Not only for her immediate health, but because truly terrible events can happen as a result of delirium.

Sally's Story

A few years ago, a woman was admitted from a D.C. hospital to a locked memory care community in Northern Virginia. She was in her late 80s and very weak.

This woman had no driver's license or any other identification when she was taken to the ER after a shopkeeper notified 911 when she was spotted stumbling outside of his store.

A 28-year-old physician then diagnosed her with dementia when she couldn't give her physical or recent history. The doctor quickly prescribed antibiotics to treat her urinary tract infection, kidney infection and pneumonia. She was given an IV to treat dehydration and, within a few days, was eating all of her meals. She quickly gained five pounds and was sent to my unit, a locked memory care floor.

Sally was pleasant and exhibited the correct social skills when I met her the Monday following her admission. Over the next two weeks, she completed her antibiotics and continued to gain weight. She politely declined to join the activities for the other residents and spent her time resting in her room. About two weeks after her admission, she met me in my office and inquired as to why she was in a secured dementia facility.

What was startling about our conversation was that she knew my name. The nature and progression of dementia means that, for the most part, by the time I meet with someone, she probably will not be able to recall my name when we meet again. (I don't generally meet people until they are in Stage Five or later.)

Secondly, Sally knew she was in a secured dementia unit, knew the address of the building, knew the date and knew her most previous history. She had no short-term memory loss and for persons with Alzheimer's, STM loss is one of the defining and first features of the disease.

As it turned out, Sally was actually Dr. Sally, a retired pediatrician. She had no living relatives and had quickly become very ill in her home. With no family members or friends to tell the ER who she was and explain her normal state, she was given a dementia diagnosis.

A mistaken diagnosis meant she had lost her apartment and her belongings. The city had claimed the apartment and her belongings had been given away. As a physician serving a poorer population, she had no savings and lived quietly and simply on her retirement. In the course of a few weeks, she had gone from living independently to living in a nursing home. No family photos, no clothing of her own, no mementoes of her life.

Sally's case is a textbook example of an ER diagnosis gone wrong. Too many times persons are given a dementia diagnosis without any actual testing for dementia other than the emergency room doctor asking an older and very sick person a series of orientation questions such as "What is your name?" or "Where are you?" or "What is today's date?" and "What is the year?"

The problem that occurs when a doctor who is not a specialist in geriatric health issues makes a dementia diagnosis in an emergency room is that some patients may actually be suffering from delirium caused by an illness.

Instead of jumping to a dementia diagnosis, the doctor should first look to determine if a fluctuating memory and reduced ability to maintain attention or shift attention appropriately has another medical cause, such as a urinary tract infection or pneumonia. Or, as in Dr. Sally's case, multiple and very serious infections.

Because delirium is not caused by long-term deterioration in the brain, its effects can be reversed with proper medical treatment.

In the end, Sally was moved to the front of the waiting list for a subsidized community in Virginia. She spent the remainder of her life living in an apartment complex that overlooked 60 acres of trees and rolling hills. Her diagnosis of dementia was removed from her record and she died peacefully in her sleep several years later.

Dementia vs. Normal Aging

One of the most common questions I am asked is how to tell the difference between dementia and normal aging, especially when we occasionally call our youngest child the name of our oldest one, can't remember the telephone number we've had for 20 years when asked for it by a sales clerk or are unable to recall where we put our car keys the evening before.

What's important to remember is that dementia is not a normal part of the aging process. It is a disease of aging, but not normal aging. Most of us will live and die experiencing only the normal forgetfulness that all human beings exhibit.

During normal aging, the body's organ systems begin to decline in function after the age of 35. These changes are slow and gradual, and the body makes adjustments throughout life to compensate for them. By the time a person reaches 60, her systems have lost 30 percent or more of their original function. Have you ever wondered why you don't collapse from your organ systems lessened functions? It is because your body started with systems that actually run above 100 percent of what you need to survive.

You probably are familiar with many of the common changes that occur. For many individuals, posture becomes more stooped; skin wrinkles and dries; and eyes lose some peripheral vision, visual clarity, depth perception and the ability to adapt to light changes. Most adults also suffer some hearing loss when the inner ear's moveable pieces become stiffer and vibrate less readily. Lungs have a decreased reserve capacity, and the heart is less able to respond to stress. Skeletons suffer a loss of bone tissue, painful arthritic changes take place in the joints and mobility is affected by a lessened ability to move quickly.

Even with all the physical changes that are a part of normal aging, the body's various systems are still quite functional into a person's 90s. Think about aging this way, a 90-year-old person is actually a person in her 10th decade of life and her body is still working!

I always thought the extra decade information was really neat. When my mother turned 70, I proudly congratulated her for making to her eighth decade of life. I thought I was delivering great news. A few years later I turned 50. I woke up feeling great and went over to my mom's for a birthday lunch. Everything was going wonderfully until she grinned an evil little grin and welcomed me to my sixth decade. Somehow, my day wasn't the same after that.

The point is as we age our brains remains fully functional with just some minor structural differences. Any changes in brain function that occur with aging more likely are related to the fact that people tend to not use their brains as much as they did when they were younger. An 80-year-old retired person probably does not read as much as when she was younger, is somewhat structured in her everyday life and simply does not challenge her brain the same way as a young adult.

In fact, the brain of an 80-year-old person is much more powerful and complex than that of a 20-year-old and not at all the stereotyped befuddled and confused elderly person portrayed on television. On the morning Dr. Sally asked me why she was in a dementia community, she named the bones in my skeleton from head to toe to prove she was alert and oriented and her brain was functioning normally. (She then asked if I would like to review the muscular structure of the human body, but I was convinced).

In the aging process, a lifetime of living experiences result in rich dendritic and neuron growth in our brains. The hemispheres of the brain begin working in a dual function after the age of 50, a process not yet fully understood. Moreover, most elderly people learn at the age of 80 at the same rate they learned at the age of 20. Given enough time to take a test, an 80-year-old woman will do just as well as she did in her younger years. Older folks may be a little slower on testing, as they are out of practice, but given enough time, their learning skills and cognition are intact.

Normal Brain Function

Dr. Ronald Devere, a board-certified neurologist and fellow of the American Academy of Neurology, says small lapses in memory – the inability to remember the name of a movie we saw two weeks ago or the need to keep a more detailed grocery list – are very common as we age, especially after we reach our late 60s. In most cases, we don't need to be especially concerned, as these small lapses normally do not interfere with our daily activities. (For more information from Devere, read his book **Memory Loss, Everything You Want To Know But Forget To Ask.**)

The fact is that normal forgetfulness can trick you into thinking that you have dementia. As you go about your day, your brain assigns value to all information around you. It is constantly reading and scanning stimuli, whether it is visual or auditory, smell, touch, light, darkness, etc. The brain is deciding what is important and what is not. That is why the noise in a restaurant or the lights in traffic or the crowd around you do not overwhelm you.

Your brain is also deciding what information you should pay attention to, for how long you should hang onto that information, what information you can ignore and what information you can dismiss as soon as the brain finishes with it.

Think about how your brain works when driving in heavy traffic. Your brain automatically assigns value to the cars around you. It decides which car needs to have your attention because that car is turning or slowing or speeding by you, and it decides which cars can be ignored at that particular time. Your brain is aware and watching for traffic lights, police, accidents and erratic drivers. As soon as the brain determines it no longer needs information for a specific car, it dismisses that information.

The same sorting of information or stimuli happens in your brain all day long. If you get up from your chair and go to another room to get something but then can't remember why you went into the other room, your brain is not demented.

Instead, it simply didn't assign value to the information. In other words, your brain didn't think what you were looking for was important enough to remember.

When you look up a telephone number and forget that number before you even dial it, chances are you are not exhibiting signs of dementia. The brain simply decided the telephone number was one you likely would never need again, so it immediately discarded the information.

And when you can't remember someone's name but can "see" the face and "feel" the name on your tongue, you likely don't have dementia. Instead, you just filed the information in a different manner than you are now attempting to access it. Think of the brain's memory like a computer.

If I once filed Brad's name in the Jennifer file and am now looking for him in Angelina's file, the computer won't be able to locate Brad. The difference between the brain and the computer, however, is that the brain will continue to try and solve the problem. This is why you will suddenly remember the name Brad at a later time.

Here's another example of how the brain looks at information: Even though you are reading this book, you likely won't remember my name. Later when a friend asks who wrote it, you won't know because my name isn't that important to your brain. What is important is the information in the book, and you'll be able to tell him some information about the history of dementia and how Alzheimer's is only one type of dementia.

If that same friend asks about your daughter Dimmy, you'll immediately be able to recall her birthday is next Saturday and she'll be 21. Your brain knows where she goes to college, the color of her car, her favorite ice cream, what she's majoring in, the name of her current beau.

So why can you remember Dimmy's birthdate, but not the birthday of the next-door neighbor, in spite having attended his birthday party? Because the information about your daughter's birthday is far more important to you, therefore your brain has a file for Dimmy's information, but not the neighbor's.

Now that you understand how a normal brain functions, also keep in mind that as a caregiver, you are more likely to read negative consequences into normal brain behavior. Because you are stressed, because you are caring for a loved one, because you have teenagers, because you are afraid of developing dementia too, you can be tricked into believing that your brain is not working properly.

If you are concerned about your brain (or your loved one's) not functioning or thinking clearly, the time to take action and insist on a proper medical evaluation is before you start to show increasingly progressive memory failures.

For example, family members or friends may find their loved one frequently asking the same questions again and again despite having been given the answer a few minutes or hours earlier. Or an individual may have regular trouble coming up with a common word or names of famous people and close family members but not be aware of the mistake.

The key point to remember is that dementia is not part of the normal aging process and should not be brushed off as such or ignored until the disease progresses to the point where a person gets lost going to the grocery store or is unable to dress appropriately. Professionals who work with the aging population believe the threshold for seeking medical attention for memory changes should be very low.

Devere says you should look at persistent memory loss the same way you would a persistent headache and seek medical attention. A diagnosis from a specialist in memory disorders (neurologist) will be helpful to an individual and family in that either 1) they are reassured there is no reason for concern, or 2) they learn the cause of memory loss is not related to dementia and is treatable, or 3) they can be proactive about preparing for a future that will be affected by dementia.

Dementia vs. Heredity

One of the most common questions I am asked by family caregivers is whether dementia is hereditary and whether they can pass the disease on to their children. Overall, most types of dementia do not appear to have a traceable hereditary pattern. Some rare forms of dementia, such as Huntington's, do have a strong genetic component. It has been suggested that some forms of Frontotemporal dementia also seems to move through the female lineage in the family, but other studies appear to point to a strong male tendency and no familial link.

For Alzheimer's, the only form that has a clear hereditary connection is the rare early onset type (EOA) where someone shows signs of the disease well before age 65. This form accounts for about three percent of Alzheimer's cases. If your loved one developed Alzheimer's after age 65, you're not necessarily pre-destined to develop the disease, though we do see some family clusters. However, studies of identical twins seem to indicate if one twin has Alzheimer's, the other twin has only a 60 percent chance of developing the disease.

In some families, we see one child in 10 with the disease; in others we see all 10 children with the disease. Some studies show that if your parent has Alzheimer's, your risk goes up 10 to 30 percent. I talk to a lot of people who insist they know someone whose great-great grandmother, great grandmother, grandmother and mother all had Alzheimer's.

However, this would be difficult to prove because when great-great grandmother and great grandmother and grandmother "had Alzheimer's," medical science simply didn't have enough knowledge about the disease process to be sure.

We also didn't have treatment for high blood pressure at that time either, so be certain to always make your physician aware of your family history. Also remember your gene package comes from your mother, so a father with dementia doesn't spell doom. Likewise, a mother's dementia has a higher impact for you, so remember to include all your family history. Don't expect the doctor to ask.

The fact is researchers do not yet completely understand the role of heredity in Alzheimer's disease. One theory is Alzheimer's is a virus lying dormant in every human that turns on in some people for some reason. Another theory is environmental triggers are behind the disease. Another is the genetics theory. And another involves the chemicals in processed foods.

What's important to know is so far researchers have not determined a clear known cause or inheritance pattern for regular or late onset Alzheimer's.

Healthy Aging for the Brain

Researchers have confirmed smoking, excessive drinking and a sedentary lifestyle are not conducive to positive aging. Smoking blocks the intact of oxygen to the brain, alcohol is technically a poison the brain must filter and a sedentary life-style means again the brain receives less oxygen. Sitting too much is now being called the new smoking, because it is recognized that humans need 150 minutes of cardiovascular activity each week.

The diet receiving the most attention at this time is the Mediterranean Diet. I don't mean that as a prescription to lie under the palm trees on a beach and sip wine, but because of its high Omega 3 fatty oils, vegetables and small amounts of red wine. Talk to your physician for more information.

Five Exercises for Your Brain

- Dancing – The brain is required to work large muscle groups in time to music and if you are dancing with a partner, your brain has to work with that complication as well.
- Games – Playing board or card games requires the brain to strategize with numbers, colors, etc. The social interaction

as you figure strategies, signals, suits, mathematical figures are great exercise for your brain.

- Playing a musical instrument – This activity requires the brain to use a completely different set of neurons and connections. (Remember, it is never too late to learn!)
- Puzzles, puzzles, puzzles! -- Any kind of word games, crosswords or number puzzles all help keep the brain firing and functioning.
- Reading – This also keeps the brain functioning at a higher level, but remember to challenge yourself with new types of literature.

＜＿＿＞

Dementia vs. Depression vs. Atypical Depression

Depression can manifest in a number of ways with dementia. It may be an illness interwoven with dementia, it may present itself in the early or mid-stages of the dementia disease process, or it may make a person appear to have dementia when she is actually suffering from depression.

In other dementias where depression is considered a probable part of the disease process, it can be dealt with through a combination of medication, cognitive therapy, increased activities and social events, and counseling depending upon the stage of the dementia.

Depression is sometimes known as pseudo-dementia because of how its symptoms mimic dementia. An elderly person who is suffering from depression, for example, is more likely to have somatic (bodily) complaints and more likely to make up illnesses or pains that are not real.

She also is more likely to become agitated and may have slower, unbalanced coordination. She may even appear to have psychotic delusions, or beliefs that are not based in reality.

It has been estimated that more than 50 percent of depression in persons with dementia suffer from is what is known as Atypical Depression. That is not a typo, it is a disease. Atypical Depression tends to present to others as the opposite of how we think of depression.

Generally, most people think of depression as an illness that might cause someone to be withdrawn, quiet, fatigued. And that would be correct – for some people. But in dementia, Atypical Depression manifests as a person with high levels of agitation, anxiety, aggression and anger. Not a person we would want to be around. Just remember, if you see these behaviors, contact your physician. Treat the behavior and seek the underlying cause of the behavior is the rule.

⌒⟶

DEPRESSION Mnemonic

The signs of depression are easier to follow if you use the letters SIGECAPS as a guide to the symptoms. In SIGECAPS, each letter in the word stands for a symptom:

S (sleep changes): An individual has an increase in day sleeping or a decreased ability to sleep at night.

I (interest): An individual shows a loss of interest in activities that used to interest her.

G (guilt): An individual doesn't place a high value on her self worth.

E (energy): An individual shows a lack of energy and often describes herself as tired or fatigued.

C (cognition and concentration): An individual appears to others as having a lessened ability to remember and think through problems and increased difficulty concentrating on tasks or daily life.

A (appetite): An individual, especially when older, may experience weight loss. Some experience weight gain, however.

P (psychomotor): An individual may appear agitated or lethargic and slow in her movements, in her relationships with others, or her thinking and recall.

S (suicide): An individual may talk about or have a sudden preoccupation with death or dying, or discuss a method she intends to try.

People over the age of sixty are more likely to have depression than any other age group. This depression tendency is the result of several reasons. One is the sense of loss. Chances are the further someone is over the age of 60, the more likely she has buried her grandparents, parents, spouse, friends and maybe even a child. For some, these losses cause an overwhelming sadness. Another reason for depression is a loss of identity.

For others, moving into an assisted living or retirement home makes them feel as though they have lost everything, including control over their lives and they are now reliant on others. Depression also can be caused by great or persistent pain, and the knowledge that a body just cannot or will not function the way it used to. Finally, most of us are fiercely independent people and who feel badly having to ask others for help or assistance with our daily tasks, even if that other person is one's own child.

But while the elderly represent only 13 percent of the population, they commit 25 percent of all suicides. The highest risk factors are living alone or feeling isolated, being male, having alcoholism, or suffering from more than one serious illness. I have even known of men in their 80s and mid-90s who committed suicide because they didn't want to "grow old and be a burden" to anyone.

If depression is present, it must be treated first. Then once the depression is under control, the person may be re-evaluated for dementia. And because so many of these outlined traits are similar to dementia, it is especially critical that a gerontology specialist be involved in the diagnosis and care process. Also understand in today's older generation, depression may not be seen as a medical problem or accepted as real.

Instead, your loved one may view depression as something suffered by lazy people and deny its existence. For this reason, a specialist will be watching for signs of depression when making a dementia assessment. In many instances, this individual will make an assessment using the Geriatric Depression Scale. This test is specifically designed to not talk about or mention depression. Instead it uses words like "blue," "down in the dumps," "tired" or "less interested" as a method of measurement that helps move past the generational stereotype for depression.

Making the Dementia Diagnosis

More often than I like to think about, I see families whose loved one was given a dementia diagnosis using nothing more than the Mini Mental Status Exam or the MMSE. Folstein and Folstein invented a short questionnaire in the 1970s known as the MMSE. The test was designed to determine a person's orientation.

The MMSE was never intended to test for a person's cognitive ability; instead its purpose is to determine if a person is alert and aware of her surroundings. Is her short-term and long-term recall working for example; is she alert and aware of her surroundings?

The questions are probably familiar to you. Is the person oriented to time, date, and place? Is her brain injured or is it functioning enough to perform basic math (what is 100 minus seven?) Who is president? What is the season?

The MMSE takes only a few minutes to give and is considered to be very reliable for deciding whether or not a person is oriented.

However, the test is not a cognition test. Cognition is very different from orientation. Although you must be oriented to pass a cognition test, it is true, the cognition test is measuring the brain's ability to function and respond to detailed questions. Look at the St. Louis University Mental Status Exam (SLUMS Test) to compare.

Instead of a math problem like "subtract the number seven from 100," the SLUMS cognition math question has more details and "thinking traps" as it were. The SLUMS Test is more like this: "If I gave you $100 and sent you to buy a tricycle for $20 and a dozen apples for $3, how much money would you spend and how much money would you have left?"

Do you see the difference? The cognition question has several numbers, a complex route for the brain to follow and used words like tri, which means three, and a dozen (12), which had nothing to do with the problem.

New cognition exams, such as this have a high validity rate of more than 96 per cent. They also detect dementia an average of five years earlier than the MMSE. Are you still guessing which test the insurance companies want used?

I once heard a neurologist describe our response to Alzheimer's in a most stunning way. He said of the 5.7 million people with

Alzheimer's in the United States, he believed only 2.5 million had been diagnosed with the disease. Of those 2.5 million persons, only 1.3 million are thought to be on medication for memory support. And sadly, he estimated that of the 1.3 million people indicated, only 600,000 were actually on the correct medication.

His shocking analysis of the current course of treatment can be attributed to three reasons: 1) Persons with Alzheimer's may not seek medical attention until the disease is quite progressed. 2) Most people are diagnosed by general practitioners and, therefore, are not necessarily being properly tested before being diagnosed. 3) A person with Alzheimer's may be prescribed incorrect (wrong dosage, wrong medication, incorrect combination of medications) or even none of the available medications for their dementia.

Although dementia cannot be stopped or reversed, certain medications have been proven to delay the progression of symptoms as well as control behavioral symptoms such as agitation, anxiety and depression. In April 2011, the National Institute of Aging released new guidelines for treating and medicating persons with any dementia. And in 2014, Devere and the State of Texas released the clinical standards to make a diagnosis.

Geriatricians, geriatric psychiatrists, and neurologists specializing in dementia are the medical specialists most likely to be aware of and prepared to follow these updates.

Medications

Currently, the U.S. Food and Drug Administration has approved three different types of cholinesterase inhibitors for persons with Alzheimer's. They are Aricept (donepezil), Exelon (rivastigmine) and Razadyne (galantamine). These three medicines prevent the breakdown of acetylcholine, a chemical in the brain believed to be related to memory, thinking and processing of information.

While it is not fully understood how these medications work, medical professionals recognize they slow the disease process for many individuals. (Still it is estimated as many as 50 percent of persons with Alzheimer's have no effect or a negative effect from the medications.) Basically, the medications allow the cells of the brain to continue to "talk" to each other by helping facilitate the neurotransmitters to make a jump across the synapses that separate cells.

When one cell "talks" to another, it releases some type of neurotransmitter across the synapse and the next cell grabs the neurotransmitter. In the next fraction of a second, enzymes go after the neurotransmitters and eat them, clearing the pathway for the next batch or firing of neurotransmitters.

As the first cell becomes sick, it begins to shrink, leaving a wider gap between the two cells. When the sick cell fires its neurotransmitters, the space between the cells is now wider. The enzymes are still waiting to gobble up the neurotransmitters, so fewer and fewer neurotransmitters are able to make the connection to the receiving cell.

These medications create fake neurotransmitters to draw off the enzymes and allow the real neurotransmitters to get through. In time, however there are too many damaged cells and the medication loses its effectiveness. As the production of acetylcholine declines, fewer and fewer healthy cells are left to talk to each other. Typically, medication is stopped in the later stages (Stages Six or Seven) of the disease.

Be aware however, once medication is stopped, your loved one will decline and restarting the medications will not bring her back to her previous level.

The other type of medication currently approved for usage is Namenda (memantine), which is designed to slow the progression of some of the symptoms of advancing dementia. Again, researchers don't quite understood how this medication works, but believe it regulates another brain chemical known as glutamate. In high amounts, glutamate is thought to accelerate brain cell death. You can expect to see a combination of these two different types of drugs being prescribed together.

Remember many dementias, like the FTDs, have no medication available at this time.

⌒

Five Points To Remember

1. Delirium is due to infection and causes rapid behavioral changes, while dementia is a slow progressing disease.

2. Dementia may or may not be inherited, but your doctor should be consulted with your concerns.

3. Delirium requires immediate medical assistance.

4. Depression can mimic dementia.

5. Medications are available to slow the disease progression in many people.

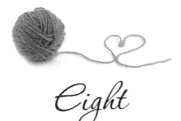

Eight

THE A'S OF DEMENTIA

As you deal with dementia, you may hear your doctor or health professional use specific medical terms – amnesia, aphasia, agnosia, and apraxia – to describe the effects of the disease. These "A's" are seen in all types of dementias, not just Alzheimer's.

Understanding the A's and their associated behaviors is important. This knowledge will allow you to provide better information to your loved one's medical professionals. Changes in your loved one's affect (how she shows emotion on her face) may be an early sign of dementia. Increased anxiety or sudden and uncharacteristic episodes of anger might be a first clue.

You may have noticed fluctuations in her ability to pay attention, an increase of agitation or an overall apathy. These first A's are subtle and can make us not want to be around our loved ones. But at the same time, they can also provide clues to the beginning and very subtle symptoms of dementia.

As dementia progresses, you will also see the amnesia, apraxia, agnosia or aphasia behaviors. In time, these A's are evident to those not familiar with your loved one.

Another reason to be familiar with the A's is that the strange, confusing and hurtful behaviors you may experience from a person with dementia will have reason and meaning. The more you're aware of these, the better able you'll be able to care for your loved one and for yourself.

As you read about the A's, keep in mind the behaviors of each "A" can be seen individually and, eventually, in conjunction with each other as their specific components begin to overlap. In other words, both amnesia and aphasia can lead to confusion about people's identity although for different reasons.

Amnesia: Inability to Use or Retain Short-Term or Long-Term Memories

Amnesia is the inability of the brain to use, make or retain short-term (new) or long-term memories. This is generally the first sign of dementia that families report noticing. Remember that regular onset Alzheimer's starts in an area at the front of the temporal lobes and the back of the frontal lobes, the two lobes that control hearing, language and smell, personality, attention, cognition, rational thought, judgment, imagination, and of course, for the Four A's, memory.

Amnesia impacts different kinds of memory, including language, procedures and life events. Amnesia is seen early in the disease process and can drive caregivers crazy.

Your loved one may forget words. One of the earliest signs in the disease process is often heard rather than seen. A mom, for example, may remember a child, but not remember the correct word to describe that child. So she may introduce her son as her husband or her daughter as her mother.

She is pulling words to describe family members from the memory file of family words, but she is getting the wrong one in spite of knowing who each child is. Perhaps you've seen when she is trying to express the need to go to the bathroom or for a drink of water, she may talk about rain or wetness. Again, she is in the file containing words for wet or water, she's just getting the wrong word.

She may repeat questions or stories. Often within minutes of hearing the answer. This can drive a caregiver crazy!

You might, for example, pick up your mother and tell her you're taking her to an appointment with the eye doctor. Five minutes later, she asks where you're taking her. You tell her again that you're driving to the eye doctor. Five minutes later, she turns to you again and asks where you are going. It is critical to remember in this early stage, your loved one will not appear to be physically ill.

She may be unable to perform tasks. Eventually amnesia causes a person to forget procedures needed to perform specific tasks, such as writing checks, cooking a meal or taking a bath. Many family members begin to realize they are facing a serious problem when they find bills unpaid or hidden away, or when a normally fastidious parent stops getting showers or washing dishes.

She may misplace belongings. Because of amnesia, the person with dementia often cannot remember where she placed items. This often results in accusations directed toward family members or caregivers such as "You stole my purse" or "You hid my keys." This type of behavior is a hallmark feature of Stage Five of the disease process.

It is hurtful and embarrassing to be accused by your own mother of stealing her car, jewelry or bank accounts. Try to understand this behavior is a result of physical damage in the brain that has changed her reality.

In your mom's world, she knows she always puts her purse on the chair by the couch. Her brain tells her she does this and she remembers doing this, but now the purse is gone. Because you are with her, her logic tells her you must have stolen her purse.

Later on when she finds the purse in the freezer, she doesn't think, "Oh I should call and apologize to my daughter." Instead she thinks something like, "What a sneaky person. Look where she hid my purse. I better hide it from her or she'll do that again."

And the cycle of losing and hiding and accusing begins anew. Understand that most families who have a loved one with dementia are hearing the same sort of accusations and that no amount of reasoning with that person will help her see the truth of the situation.

She may lack sound decision-making abilities. Memory lapses can cause poor decisions. Alzheimer's people simply forget that they are not allowed to drive a car or that they must turn off the stove after making a grilled cheese sandwich.

Even though she looked sincere and was truly sincere when she promised not to drive the car or turn on the stove, her damaged brain didn't take in and hold onto the new information. What her brain remembers is she can drive a car, because she's been driving a car for decades. Or she knows how to safely cook food. She may give away large sums of money to family members or strangers. (Be aware this can happen in person, via mail or over the Internet.)

Keep in mind memories are typically lost in the reverse order of how they were formed, as explained in Chapter 5. This is why recently learned information – someone's short-term memory – goes away first and why a normally organized mother continues to ask the same question over and over. She may insist she wasn't given breakfast even though she ate a stack of pancakes five minutes ago.

This inability to form new memories is why she gets mad she wasn't told about the family gathering for a birthday or forgets where she put her keys and accuses her husband, children or caregiver of hiding them.

⁓

The Colonel's Story

One spring day, I was bringing a retired Air Force colonel I had known for quite a while back to his home following a doctor's visit. We had a 45-minute drive ahead when he turned to me and asked, "So are you married?"

I explained I was married to a retired Army colonel. When he asked if I had any children, I told him I did not but had a couple of dogs. He then asked if we had ever been posted to the Pentagon. I explained my spouse had retired from the Pentagon before we'd moved to Texas. He made a comment about the "lovely day" and then turned to look out the window at the lake and vividly colored wildflowers.

He and I were having a perfectly appropriate social conversation. But then just a few seconds later, he turned to me again. "So are you married?" he asked. Without skipping a beat, we repeated the entire conversation five more times. As I answered the same questions over and over, I couldn't help but think about how confusing or annoying this conversation would be for someone who didn't understand Alzheimer's.

The colonel didn't look sick. He could have been anybody's grandfather. With his white hair and erect posture and gripping handshake, his eyes always twinkled when we met. The gentleman wasn't trying to be difficult. He was just enjoying a conversation with me.

His social skills were deeply embedded in older memory files, so he was perfectly capable of displaying those well-practiced social skills. However, the damage in his brain didn't allow him to record and remember the conversation because his hippocampus (the part of the brain used to form new memories) was damaged.

⌐

Using the Files

Eventually the Alzheimer's person will turn to older memories, such as those from childhood or young adulthood memories, to fill in gaps in the current memory. This explains why a mom who doesn't remember where she has lived for the past 40 years asks to go to a home. She's looking for that particular home where she grew up because those are the memories her brain is now using.

When she looks around at her current home, she doesn't recognize it. Instead her brain remembers her parents' home is located in the small town of Pearl, Texas. And that's where her brain tells her she needs to go. This is a common occurrence when a person is moved into a community, or when you move your loved one in with you.

You'll find many residents or your mom continually requesting to go home. She may tell you it is because her mom and dad are waiting for her, she needs to cook for her children, or she has to go to work. This happens despite the fact her "home" no longer exists except in her mind (and heart).

Amnesia's reverse chronological memory loss pattern also helps explain why the youngest child may be forgotten first while memories of the oldest child remain. (This is not true for all dementia patients as some retain the memories of all their children). In some cases, a parent who doesn't recognize her own children may refer to them by the names of relative – a father, mother, sister or brother; a cousin, aunt or uncle – who that child resembles.

What is happening is her brain is drawing on a familiar facial features that make individuals from one family tend to resemble each other. When your mom doesn't recognize you, your file is damaged or gone. However, because your resemblance to her sister remains, her brain says you must be that sister.

We all carry our family features. Some genetic characteristics are stronger than others, but they are there. For example, if you looked at all my nieces and nephews, you would be able to tell they are related. They are the products of my four siblings, but they all have similar features.

Even adopted children resemble their families, through facial or body postures, verbal pronunciations, etc. These subtle ways of movement or faces may no longer exist in your file, but they are in a file somewhere, so you become that person.

Without a doubt, amnesia behaviors are confusing and stressful for family members, especially because dementia doesn't cause anyone to look sick in the early and middle stages. Also, in the beginning stages of the disease, the memory can be slippery. Sometimes she can grasp it completely, and sometimes she can only use a portion of it. One consequence of these behaviors is that family caregivers can easily lose patience and snap at their loved one because it seems as though she is doing these annoying behaviors on purpose.

However, if you look at memory loss through the eyes of the person with Alzheimer's, you can envision how confusing life can be. Imagine being told over and over that the strange woman with the gray hair is your daughter when, in your mind, you work at the war department and never married. Or imagine thinking that your husband has turned into a sneaky, mean and spiteful man who continually hides your slippers and newspaper.

Her Reality Is Your Reality

Unfortunately, trying to correct amnesia creates greater confusion and paranoia for your loved one, and may lead to outbursts or aggression if she becomes convinced you are lying. This means the best way to deal with amnesia behaviors is not to correct the individual or to try to get her to remember. This is hard to do because as humans we are natural teachers who have correct mistakes. Think about the thousand times you corrected your child's speech, or said, "No do it this way," when explaining something.

In caring for a person with dementia, you need to go along with her perceptions and memories by understanding that her reality must become your reality. We used to believe that we cold reorient a person to reality if we just repeated it enough. So every morning, in every community, the activity department or the caregiver would say the day's date, year, president, month, week and so forth.

But what we began to understand was insisting to a lady who thinks the year is 1942 and she is single, that the year is 2013 and she is a great-grandmother not only scares her, but it also makes her paranoid. Imagine if right now all the people around you began to insist the year was 2030. You would wonder what was wrong with you that you didn't know the correct year, or you might decide to stay away from those "crazy" people.

If your mom asks for the salt and you know she meant the sugar, just hand her the sugar. Instead of insisting to Mom she was actually invited to the birthday party but forgot, just move on. If she can't find her purse, but you find it in the cupboard with the cereal, don't berate her for putting it in the wrong place. Just hand her the purse. If she inquires about where you found it, just tell her you found it.

But Dad Is Dead!

Dealing with memory loss when it involves people who have already died is especially challenging. If a wife is looking for her husband who actually died 10 years ago, don't tell her he's dead. Being told that someone you love is dead is devastating the first time it is heard and constantly correcting your loved one about the status of the person she is looking for is cruel, as it forces her to relive that moment of grief each time she hears the news.

Some families may respond to a person's search for a deceased loved one by using "therapeutic lying," where they tell that person that her husband is not home and at a logical place such as work or the golf course. If you do this, however, be prepared for an outburst if she demands to go there and find him.

Be prepared for the consequences when you decide to try this for yourself. I have received too many midnight calls because someone decided he or she had to tell a person with dementia the truth about a loved one's death. The result can be contacting your doctor for medication to calm your loved one down. It can mean watching in horror as she relives the memory over and over for days or weeks or months. It can mean being shocked when she doesn't know who you are telling her about.

A better method is to try to listen to her feelings when she talks about a deceased loved one and steer the conversation in a different direction. Look at a photo of the person, ask about when they met or other significant events, and gradually move her away from the topic of the person and onto a different subject.

This method of dealing with a loved one with dementia is challenging and takes time, but is an ethical and safe way to help her through a powerful memory. Although this skill of validating feelings can be painful for you, it also may prove to be healing. As you guide your loved one through her fears in a world that no longer makes sense to her, the process can also lead to powerful and poignant memories that may give you unexpected gems and carry you through the next round of challenges.

Aphasia: Inability to Use or Understand Language

The second "A" of dementia is aphasia, or the inability to use and understand language. This gradual loss of communications skills takes place as the temporal lobes are attacked and damaged. Aphasia will begin to overlap with amnesia because memory, speech, language and hearing are closely linked. The left lobe of the brain contains words and name memories while the right side holds pictures and faces, all key objects we need to recall and use language.

The level of language loss depends up the stage of the disease. In the early stages, you may just see occasional word substitutions of related words, such as using the word "son" when referring to a husband or the word "coffee" when talking about tea. Or similar sounding words may be interchanged, such as the use of "bat" instead of "hat." These so-called slips of the tongue happen to everyone occasionally. Only when they become regular occurrences should a family begin to suspect a problem related to dementia.

As the disease progresses, additional language problems will surface, and a person's speech will grow more confusing and difficult to follow. For example, instead of substituting a related word, the person may begin to use an unrelated or unintelligible word. Pronunciations may be incorrect or words may run together. And as someone has more difficulties retrieving correct words, she may start to use vague terminology like "whatchamacallit" or else launch into a lengthy description of an item to substitute for a loss of vocabulary fluency. "You know, that thing, you know we use it to you know, that thing."

Toward the later stages of the disease, expect a lot of repetition of words or phrases. Eventually, the Alzheimer's person will be unable to follow simple directions or even express that she is hurt, sick or hungry. And you can anticipate a loved one who speaks more than one language to revert to her original one, as these files of her first language have existed longer in her memory.

If you don't know your mother's native language, you will need to prepare a communication book of common words such as bathroom, water, thirsty, doctor, pain and hungry. If your mother is in a community and no caregivers speak her language, the facility will need a book as well. I was once in a dementia community in Virginia where 10 separate language books were being used by the staff to communicate with its diverse residents.

Finally, in the end stage of dementia, a person will be unable to use or understand any language, either written or spoken.

Aphasia behaviors can be frustrating for families. Early in the disease, an Alzheimer's person will laugh off mistake, deny she made one, or simply nod and pretend to understand. As language skills deteriorate more and the capacity to communicate plummets, you'll find it even more difficult to meet your loved one's needs.

What's important to remember is this is not happening because your loved one is being absentminded, stubborn, stupid or cruel. Instead, her brain is under attack and she cannot help, or stop, her increasing confusion.

Many families have difficulty understanding the extreme loss of language a person with dementia suffers. Because the person doesn't look sick, because the automatic "yes/no" speech is still functioning, or because you love this person very much, her language loss can be hard to accept. Once the subtle changes in the use of language occur with speech, the person is also having difficult understanding what is being said.

I tested a man once who wife insisted he understood at least 90 percent of what she was saying. The test indicated a rate of about 30 percent. Imagine how angry she was with him at times because he didn't response to her or do what she had asked? He wasn't trying to be difficult; his brain just didn't understand the words.

To accommodate the changes in language abilities caused by aphasia, family members and caregivers will have to adjust how they communicate as the disease progresses. Chapter 8 of this book is dedicated to dealing communication issues throughout the course of dementia and provides tips about how you can accommodate these challenges.

John's Story

man I know was struggling with his mother's advancing dementia. She had been a bright and vigorous little woman until being diagnosed with Progressive Aphasic Dementia, a lesser-seen Frontotemporal Dementia that causes significant damage to the lobes of the brain involved with memory, speech and language.

After years of the disease, she had little speech or language abilities left, and had not spoken a complete, coherent sentence in months.

One day John was confronted with a tearful, flustered mother whose language loss kept her from telling him why she was perturbed. Not only was John was at a loss of what to do and how to comfort his mother; he harbored great guilt about his mother's disease.

As a younger man, John had struggled with addiction. He had been lost to his family over the years and the overwhelming loss of his mother to dementia threatened to stop him from ever making his apologies.

Because John's mom was in an assisted living community, he could have easily alerted the staff to his mother's condition and left the building. Nonetheless, as she struggled that day with her agitation, John remained near in her room. When she allowed it, he began to pat her hand. He spoke soothingly to her and told her repeatedly how much he loved her.

As she calmed, John began to pour out his heart to her. He told how sorry he was she was upset and how he wished he could help her as she had so often helped him. John told her he loved her for being his mother and how he wished he had gotten sober before the disease had taken her away. John sobbed as he apologized for the hurt and pain he had brought to the family and for the years he had stayed away.

John's mother, who had calmed down by this point, held tightly to his hand and looked squarely at his face and said, "I thought of you always."

That was the last complete sentence she ever spoke. The following year as she lay dying, John and his sister Mary stayed by her side. "I thought of you always" became the final powerful memory John kept of his mother.

Agnosia: Inability to Recognize Common Objects or People

Agnosia takes place as the frontal, occipital and temporal lobes of the brain become damaged. Behaviors associated with this

"A" mean the brain develops an inability to recognize and use common everyday objects.

One example that illustrates the confusion between common objects is mistaking a toothbrush for a hairbrush. The brain may become confused because both items are brushes, or because both brushes are found in the bathroom. Maybe it is because both have handles and bristles and they are used for something around the head area.

Think about pens and pencils. These are easily confused too. Each instrument is held in the hand and each leaves marks on paper. Although this may not seem like much of a problem, the difference between signing a check with a pen and signing a check with a pencil can be costly.

Every day, without even thinking about it, we use a variety of objects to accomplish everything from cleaning and grooming to cooking and eating and more. Gradually, the ability of how to use these tools is lost by changes in the brain. The files are destroyed.

Take eating utensils, for instance. As an infant and then young child, you were fed liquids and then pureed food. As your coordination got better and your chewing skills developed, you were given finger foods or began to learn how to use a spoon. After the spoon, you began to use a fork, and finally a fork and knife.

As dementia progresses, your loved one will take this journey again, but in the reverse order. She will go from knowing how to use a fork and knife to knowing only how to use only a fork. She will then use a spoon, but eventually she will forget how to use utensils completely and will start eating with her hands. Near the end of the disease, she will have to be fed by a caregiver.

As dementia progresses, she will also become lost in familiar places. When this occurs, she will have difficulty recognizing rooms in her home, such as a bathroom, or the purpose of those rooms. She may not be able to find her way from her home to the store. She may get lost in the town where she has lived for decades.

She will probably have difficulty recognizing family members and other people she once knew. What we're talking about here goes beyond the memory lapses of amnesia.

With agnosia, the Alzheimer's brain has lost its ability to translate what the eyes see or to find the file that contains information about a person, making it impossible to determine if someone is familiar. In the later stages, many dementia patients do not recognize any family members or even themselves.

Remember Martha who didn't remember getting married or having a daughter? When she looked in the mirror, she became alarmed about the old lady in her bathroom. In actuality, the old lady was Martha. However, because her brain was using files from when she was only 24 years old, she no longer recognized herself. It is not unusual for an affected person to refuse to go into the bathroom because someone is already there. Or you may witness her having a conversation with the person in the mirror or getting annoyed with the stranger in the window who refuses to talk to her.

How Would You Feel?

The problems caused by the A's can cause extreme anxiety for those who suffer from dementia. Imagine how frightening the world would be if you could not recognize food items, a toothbrush or toilet, clothing, a vacuum or stove, or rooms in your own home.

Imagine how frightening the world would be if you suddenly realized when out on a walk or drive that you had no idea where you were or how to get to safely home. Can you imagine how scary the world would be if people you no longer recognized regularly appeared in your house and tried to make you eat food or take a bath or change your clothes?

As difficult as it is, you must understand when someone doesn't get recognize an object such as a toilet, or a person as important as her own husband or child, that person is not pretending or being stubborn. Instead of getting frustrated or mad, you'll need to try and find a way around the problem. For object and rooms, you might try putting labels on objects and rooms, though this will only work for a while.

Dealing with the inability to recognize people, however, is more complicated. If someone you didn't know suddenly appeared in your house, you would be frightened. You might try to fight off the stranger or you might scream for help. Chances are you would want the police to assist you.

It is not uncommon to hear reports about physical altercations between spouses when a wife doesn't recognize her husband and starts beating the so-called home invader with a broom, or when a husband physically pushes his wife out of the house because he didn't recognize the person in his bedroom as the woman he has been married to for many years.

Interestingly, while a woman has been trained throughout life to call out for help or protect herself physically when discovering a stranger in her home, a man faced with the discovery of a strange woman in his house usually has a different response.

Oftentimes he will remember being married, but doesn't recognize this woman as his wife. What he does know is he had better get this new woman out of his house before his "real" wife gets home or he'll have "hell to pay." This socialization of the sexes means wives can be at risk to be physically hurt by husbands and vice versa. In addition to the physical pain, it is also very difficult to have your spouse not recognize you. It can be heartbreaking.

Conversation Tips

One way to try and deal with people recognition problems is to give a person clues that may help her brain make some sort of connection. For example, you might start a conversation with your mom something along the lines of this: "Here's a picture of dad and me from when we visited the Grand Canyon. I'm your daughter Terria, and I remember standing on the edge of the canyon while you took pictures. Wow did you yell at me to get away from the edge!"

Or, "Hi Mom, I'm your daughter Mary Ann. I'm your baby. You have always loved me more than your other children! You always said I'm the prettiest!"

With this type of greeting, you have given your loved one a variety of social and memory clues, such as your name, a reminder of her husband, a memory about a trip, or a laugh from how she fussed at you or teased you.

This sort of social greeting is much more appropriate than starting a conversation with "Do you know who I am?" or "What's my name?" or any other number of questions that challenge the person with dementia.

Two things are wrong with this approach. First, the person is already burdened by trying to make sense of a confusing world. Directing questions toward someone who cannot answer them because of damage to her brain by dementia just adds to the confusion. It increases paranoia and can increase verbal or physical agitation as a result. Remember suspicion is also a part of dementia.

Second, social skills function until late in the disease, that is, they are deep in the file cabinet. Not being able to answer questions like "Hey do you know who I am?" is embarrassing and humiliating. Those feelings can cause a person to withdraw further. Think about how you feel when you've bumped into someone you've met before but could not remember his or her name.

Chances are you were you embarrassed and frustrated while you tried to pretend you knew that person. Meanwhile, your brain was frantically searching for the information you needed about that person. Someone with dementia experiences these same feelings over and over, until that too is lost.

Apraxia: Inability to Use Coordinated and Purposeful Movement

When your loved one is unable to carry out a routine motor tasks, such as turning on the TV, tying her shoelaces, brushing her teeth, moving in and out of a chair, walking or standing and turning, chewing or swallowing food or controlling her bladder or bowel, in spite of the fact that she the physical capacity and the desire, she is now experiencing the effects of apraxia.

Medically speaking, apraxia is the inability of the prefrontal motor cortex and the parietal lobes of the brain to coordinate purposeful movement. In other words, both the lower and upper parts of the brain that integrate the information needed to perform movements are deteriorating and no longer able to send movement signals to the muscles. This causes a type of disconnect between the idea of a task and the execution of the task.

Signs of apraxia also signal that Alzheimer's is completing its circular route through the brain and has left its mark in the front (frontal lobes), back (occipital lobes), bottom (temporal lobes) and top (parietal lobes) areas.

You see apraxia when someone picks up a glass of juice and is unable to move it to her mouth. Fine coordinated hand movement is lost. Instead, she may pour her drink onto the table or in her plate of food. She may even be unable to hold the glass at all. Likewise, she may grab onto something, like a glass or a caregiver's wrist, with more intensity then needed and then be unable to let go or release her grip.

Apraxia also impacts a brain's ability to tell the body how to stay in balance while standing, walking or sitting.

Falls and Dementia

One consequence of damage to the parts of the brain that control movement is that a person's risk for falls (and injury from falls) becomes a real concern. When added to continuing deterioration of the occipital lobe and resulting loss of peripheral vision and depth perception, a person's gait will begin to change. Steps become shorter and eventually she may not lift her feet from the floor at all as she moves.

As the brain is damaged from dementia, the person cannot safely maneuver. Trying to force her to stand when she says she can't only increases the risk of falling, except now you may get hurt as well if she falls with you. Falls are not a sign of poor care; they are an indicator of infection, delirium, or the progression of the disease.

Remember, even if a person knew how to walk this morning or just a moment ago, because her brain can't find the right pathway of signals, she may not be able to walk in this moment. Accusing her of "faking" her abilities is cruel. People with dementia are doing the best they can every moment of the day. They don't, in spite of how it may appear, have the ability to pretend or fake a behavior.

Falls are a part of the disease. They are scary and can cause bruising to the brain (hematomas or contusions). Falls can be deadly because of the impact of the head on the floor. Seizures, stroke activity, internal bleeds, double vision and an increase in amnesia can all result from a fall.

Remember as the disease progresses, the brain structure inside the cranium is smaller. When the head strikes the floor, for example, the whiplash effect means the brain is actually bouncing inside the cranium from the front to the back, a double blow known as contra coup trauma.

Broken hips can result from a fall or may trigger the fall. Let me explain. When people with advanced dementia stand, they may turn suddenly, causing the body to twist at the hips. Frail and fragile bones can literally snap below the ball joint, resulting in a "twist and turn" fracture. The person then falls and the appearance or common belief is that the fall resulted in a broken hip. In reality, the broken hip resulted in the fall.

It is not unusual for some hip fractures to not be repaired. Your surgeon will discuss with you whether or not your loved one is a good candidate for surgery or any other risk factor. Just keep in mind that people with dementia do not come out of surgery the same. There is typically a marked decline in abilities, often quite noticeable to families. Their brains don't recover from anesthesia the same way you and I would.

In the end, falls are a sign the body is starting to fail, not that the caregivers aren't being responsive. The real trick as it were, is to get your loved one from a walking to a happily sitting person. Most families are plagued by how to keep an unsafe person in a chair and not constantly trying to stand and attempt to walk. Since restraints aren't legal in most states, families use chair alarms, pillows or stuffed animals to keep in the person's lap and hopefully keep her sitting safely.

In Stage Six, her step will become a small two- to three-inch movement forward, a shuffling movement she can keep at for hours, even past the point of exhaustion.

In time, apraxia affects all muscular movement. Facial features will become flatter as the brain will not be able to send signals to the face to make the subtle movements that are interpreted by professionals as "affect." A person also slowly loses the ability to perform any of her activities of daily living, i.e., sleeping, ambulating (walking), toileting, grooming, hygiene care, dressing, eating. This means her physical capabilities, along with her mental capabilities will transition from those of an adult, to those of a child, to those of a newborn baby.

Near the end of the disease process, the brain is so damaged that the devastating loss of ability to use muscular structure means your loved one will be unable to walk, sit, hold up her head, or chew or swallow food safely. This profound loss of ability means your loved one will need total care and supervision during the final stages of the disease.

The A's Mix Up

The A's tend to follow the order of amnesia, aphasia, agnosia and apraxia because of how the disease is moving through the brain. Just remember one "A" does not go away when another "A" starts.

Instead, they begin to overlap and occur together. Remember the earlier example of a misplaced purse that ended up in the freezer? Amnesia caused mom to forget where she put her purse. The reason the purse ended up in the freezer was a result of agnosia because she didn't recognize the purse as a purse at that particular time nor did she recognize that the refrigerator as the wrong place to store a purse.

Lorraine's Story

Lorraine became an agitated and anxious lady as dementia worked its course. She had been married to a career Air Force colonel. A widow for 20 years, she had never remarried. Her husband's photo, a beaming young man in uniform standing next to his newly married wife, sat next to her bed. It was the first thing she looked at each morning and the last thing she touched each night. Lorraine also had been a successful clothing buyer for a large department store chain.

One day she came to my office and after several minutes and much effort on her part to speak, I figured out she was missing a pair of pants. Because I knew she had been a clothing buyer, I thought I could figure out what pair of pants she was missing by naming every type of material I could think of. Sounds like a good plan, right?

I asked her if she was missing her wool pants and she shook her head 'No." I asked about her corduroy, silk and knit pants. Again, she shook her head "no" each time. I asked her if she was looking for dungarees (people from Lorraine's generation didn't wear blue jeans; they wore dungarees).

Her struggle to speak resulted mostly in gibberish until she finally was able to blurt out, "Army pants! My army pants!"

Did you figure out which pair of slacks she was looking for yet? During World War II, the military wore khaki uniforms. Lorraine's files in her brain were full of military information. Part of the files existed because she lived through WWII and part of her files had khaki pants because her husband was a career officer.

I opened her closet door, which required pulling the handle towards me and slightly to the left and looked in the dirty clothes hamper. There they were. Lorraine literally clapped her hands with glee when she saw the pants.

Lorraine's story shows us how the A's will overlap as Alzheimer's progresses. When Lorraine couldn't remember where her pants were, she was suffering from amnesia. When she couldn't find the words to say she was trying to find her khaki pants, she experienced aphasia. When she didn't recognize the pants must be in the dirty clothes hamper or know what the hamper was, agnosia was at work. Apraxia meant she couldn't perform the movements required open the closet door.

The brain's processing of information through the course of amnesia, aphasia, agnosia and apraxia is difficult and challenging for caregivers. Think of the inability to remember a word (amnesia) and the inability to understand a word (aphasia) or the inability to recognize a fork as a fork (agnosia) and an inability to use it properly (apraxia).

Dementia Behaviors Appear Random

Another reason dementia behaviors are tough is they seemingly come and go with no particular pattern as the brain works to find – sometimes successfully – alternate pathways to process information.

For example, your mom may not recognize you for several days in a row and then, out of the blue, call you by name and ask about her grandchildren by name. Then the next day, she's back to referring to you as her mother. This back and forth is extremely hard on families and caregivers, especially because they never know exactly when the alternate pathways will succumb to the disease and the ability for their loved ones to recognize them will be gone for good.

Occasional blips of vacancy you saw in your mother's eyes in the beginning eventually become the norm as moments of clarity become farther and farther apart.

Coming to terms with the disease is difficult, especially in the beginning and middle stages, because the afflicted person simply does not look ill and may have no obvious physical impairments. When a husband has a stroke and loses the ability to use his right arm and leg, a wife or child understands and can see why he cannot feed himself. When a grandmother is diagnosed with macular degeneration and her visual acuity is impaired, we accept that she cannot see her grandchildren and, therefore, forgive her for not recognizing them when they walk into the room.

With Alzheimer's and the other dementias, the limbs remain strong and the eyes are able to see. The damage taking place in the brain is not visible to us, thus making our leap to understanding behaviors all that more difficult. For this reason, try to cherish the good moments and recognize the challenging ones as the disease and not your loved one.

So let's add one more big "A." **Anosognosia** is the inability to recognize impaired function in memory, general thinking skills, emotions and body functions. This means your loved one really doesn't remember (not denial) she has dementia. As the disease progresses she doesn't remember that she has a brain illness.

Six Points to Remember

1. Amnesia is the inability to use or retain short- or long-term memory.

2. Aphasia is the inability to use or understand language.

3. Agnosia is the inability to recognize or use common objects or people.

4. Apraxia is the inability to use coordinated and purposeful movement.

5. Anosognosia is the inability to recognize impaired function in memory, general thinking skills, emotions and body functions.

6. Understanding the A's helps us understand and better cope with the behaviors seen in people with dementia.

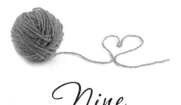

Nine

Changes in the Five Senses

To successfully function as a human, your brain must be able to constantly recognize stimuli, filter them and make correct interpretations about what's happening in your physical and social environment. A healthy brain is so adept at this process that you usually don't even realize it is happening.

For example, as you read this chapter, chances are a number of other sounds may be taking place near you. A show may be on the television, the air conditioning may be cycling on and off, a door may bang closed, someone may be talking on the phone, a dog outside may be barking and so on.

A correctly working brain pays attention to the important sounds and ignores the less important ones. This is why you don't notice the sound of a fan but do notice the sound of a ringing doorbell or honking horn. In other words, your brain is assigning value to the stimuli around you and deciding what is important and what can be ignored as background noise.

The same concept applies to what you see and feel. Your brain determines if the ground your eyes perceive in front of you is safe or the dangerous edge of a cliff. Your brain determines if the air temperature is too hot or too cold so you can decide whether to put on or take off a sweater.

When a person has dementia, physical changes in the brain severely impact its ability to understand, hear, recognize or sort external stimuli. This means that individual's ability to comprehend her environment gradually fades until it is completely gone, making an already complex world seem even more complex, confusing and dangerous.

Not only will her brain eventually lose the ability to understand and identify noises, but it also will be unable to interpret what the eyes see, the taste buds taste or the skin feels.

By understanding these changes in perception and accommodating the diminishing ability to make sense of surroundings, caregivers and family members are able to provide a safer physical environment, better emotional care and a less complex day-to-day structure for a person with dementia – all important ways to make that individual's world easier to navigate and understand.

Interpreting Sight

When dementia begins to destroy the brain's occipital lobe, the ability of the eye itself is not damaged. Instead, the part of the brain that controls or interprets what the eye sees is damaged. If you feel the back of your head, the occipital lobe is located at the bottom and back of your skull just above your neck.

As the disease progresses, a person with Alzheimer's will experience subtle and gradual changes in her depth and distance perception. This means her view of the world changes from a normal three-dimensional one to a flatter one-dimensional interpretation. In other words, the world begins to looks more and more like a photograph as the concept of distance loses meaning.

This causes great difficulty for the person to judge distance as well as the location of one item in relation to another item. The result is more bumping into doorways, desks, chairs, couches and tables as well as the frequent misses when reaching for items. The individual may have difficulty catching a ball or clapping her hands.

I have visited memory communities where depth perception changes were readily evident in a fairly common group activity meant to be fun way to provide exercise and engagement with peers. But in reality it was a frightening experience for some participants.

In this game, the activity person bounces a ball to a semi-circle of residents. The residents are supposed to catch the ball and then throw or bounce the ball back to the activity person. Inevitably, one or more residents jump fearfully when the ball is bounced towards them.

Not only does the ball sometimes come toward the resident at a speed that her brain cannot comprehend, she also is not able to determine the depth relationship of the ball at its starting point. Because her damaged brain takes longer to translate any movement, she jumps in fear each time the ball is passed to her.

A friendly game of bounce becomes a terrifying game of dodge ball. (Changing the ball from a hard ball to a beach ball can help this resident as a beach ball moves slower, isn't as hard and is easy to "swat" away).

Depth Perception Changes

Another common problem caused by depth perception changes has to do with how a person with dementia perceives the ground where she is walking. You may have no problem stepping from carpeting to a wood or tile floor. To a person with dementia, however, a shiny, waxed floor may appear to be shimmering water or seem as though it is moving.

Remember the last time you walked into a public bathroom with the orange cones announcing wet floors? Did you stride in confidently or carefully place each step?

Where you may move from a light colored sidewalk to a black asphalt street easily and without fear, for the person with dementia, the dark asphalt may be perceived as a deep hole. Depth perception problems also cause fear with steps and staircases.

For all these reasons, it is not unusual to see a person with dementia tapping the floor with her foot as she tests where she's about to step as she moves into a new area or steps onto an elevator. She is doing this because she can't be certain she's stepping onto a stable surface.

Peripheral Vision

As someone enters the later stages of the disease process, peripheral vision also becomes severely impaired. This means the Alzheimer's person no longer sees or interprets visual clues that come from the side. In other words, approaching her from a direction other than the front means she can be easily startled. You may appear to seemingly jump out of nowhere.

Try it like this: Imagine if you were walking down the hallway to your kitchen alone in your home and someone suddenly jumped out next to you. Chances are you would instinctively swing at whatever scared you as you tried to protect yourself from danger or harm.

This same reflexive action, the instinctual response inherent in each of us, designed to protect one's self and survive, remains strong even in those with dementia. In many cases where I've been asked to assess a combative person with dementia who was swinging at and striking caregivers, I've found that a loss of peripheral vision and the resulting startle reaction was causing the outbursts. The incorrect approach of the caregiver was the cause of a reflexive and protective action.

Another consequence of peripheral vision loss can be seen in eating patterns. A person with Alzheimer's may eat food only from one side of a plate or in an area that's shaped like of a wedge of pie. This is not a sign that the individual only loves potatoes and nothing else; instead, it is a sign that she can only see a portion of the plate. If someone is eating from only one part of her plate, simply continue to rotate the plate to allow her to see more of the food.

Telescope Vision

You also may see individuals towards the end of the disease process reach out and "pinch" the air in front of them. This picking or pinching in the air is related to the brain's inability to focus and translate what it is seeing. In other words, the individual is trying to touch objects that are not actually in front of her.

To get an idea of her visual abilities at this stage, shut one eye and place your curled up hand around your other eye. Your fingertips should be along the side of your thumb, creating a tunnel for the eye to peer through. This will give you a fairly accurate concept of how someone with dementia is seeing the environment around her. Is there any wonder she is easily startled or scared?

Look around you now. Can you see your plate of food directly under your nose? Can you see the food across the table? Which one would you reach for? Remember at this point, impulse control is damaged, so you don't think you are taking your neighbor's food or dessert.

As you think about vision challenges that come with dementia, always try to imagine how these changes impact your loved one. For example, if your mom is living in a memory or assisted living community, remember that when she looks down a hallway, she is not seeing or interpreting that hallway the same way as you and I. We see a hallway that makes sense. We know that different rooms are located along the hallway, and we can judge the distance between the rooms and the length of the hallway.

However, to your mom, the hallway may look long and empty with no clues to make sense of the space. It may appear to go on forever. Hallways and rooms in communities generally painted bland colors with few or no decorations allowed on the outside of the doors. Some communities will insist that small changes they make in door trim will assist your loved one in locating her room. Take this theory with a grain of salt and keep in mind that your loved one sees a white door, not a small piece of white trim on a white door.

More typically, the only distinguishing door marks are small room numbers and possibly a small photo of the room's resident. If a photo is present, it is posted for two reasons. One is to help staff recognize the person and make certain that person is the correct one when it comes time to administer medication. The second reason is that well meaning people think the photo will help your mother identify a specific room as hers.

This second reason is the one that makes the least sense in most cases. Remember, based on the stage of the disease, your mom may or may not recognize her own picture. Also, for an elderly person, or anyone over 40 for that matter, the ability to see small objects has diminished with age. A face in a photograph is usually the size of a dime or smaller.

Add dementia-caused damage to vision in the occipital lobes and lost memory files in the frontal lobes, and being able to interpret the meaning of the photo is lost. Moreover, these photos and room numbers are usually located about 70 inches above the floor despite the fact that many residents may be in wheelchairs or simply not tall enough to see the identifying numbers or photo.

⟜⟶

Memory Box

Another common identifying door marker is a photo or memory box. Family members are instructed to add photos and mementos to this box to help their loved one locate her room. For the reasons explained in the previous section, this usually doesn't do much good for the resident.

If you do have an opportunity to put one together however, go ahead. These types of boxes have a positive psychological impact on the caregiving staff. Because families place photos and memorabilia of the resident at different times of her life, caregivers see that individual as more than simply a demented resident.

Instead, the photos will help them remember that your mother was once a little girl, a teenager, a bride, a young wife, a young mother, a grandmother or great-grandmother. Prompting more life stage connections will unconsciously assist the caregiver in viewing your mom as a whole human being and not just an old woman who may have unpleasant behaviors or require a higher level of care.

One of the best photo boxes I've seen is in a community in Round Rock, Texas. There the owners put the frame for a box in the center of the door and made it large. The activity department helps families place photos from different ages of the person on bright backgrounds of red, blue, yellow, green, etc.

Doing a photo box this way is very helpful to the person with dementia. She may not recognize the tiny photos, but she can see the bright colors and identify her room.

Here are some additional tips to help cope with changes in visual perception:

- Move more slowly and deliberately around people with dementia to give their brains time to process information. The rule is one-step for one second.

- Ensure pathways are clear by taking up all rugs and other types of clutter that could cause trips. Look for and remove other smaller items such as footstools, home décor and unworn shoes that could cause trips or falls. Remember, most falls occur in the bathroom and kitchen because these two rooms are most likely to have small rugs and wet or greasy surfaces. Arrange furniture in a way that the backs of sofas and chairs can be used as handrails as someone moves around a room.

- If you are worried about your mom falling out of her bed or attempting to get out of her chair, you can order a bed or chair alarm. These alarms are commonly used in facilities because it is illegal to belt, tie or restrain a person in a chair or bed.

- When approaching someone with dementia from behind, walk around the person at arm's length and tell her you are coming around her. Touch her on the shoulder while you are talking to help her gauge where you are and to associate your voice with the person who "suddenly" appears at her side. Remember one step for each second.

- If allowed, use bright name signs and other decorations in colors that elderly people more easily see (red or purple is better than pastels) to help make a room entrance or door look more distinctive and identifiable. Make sure these signs and decorations are placed at the person's actual eye level.

Interpreting Taste and Smell

Most people lose taste buds as they age and have a lessened ability to taste their food. This is different than the loss of taste that affects Alzheimer's people. What happens to them is that they gradually lose their ability to perceive almost any taste except for sweet. Think about it like this. If your favorite meal was steak and I prepared you a beautiful steak, but when you took a bite your brain perceived the flavor of the steak as something more like cardboard. Chances are that you wouldn't eat much of it.

But if I put ketchup or barbecue sauce or brown sugar or syrup, etc., on the steak, your brain receives the flavor as tasty and you get to enjoy your steak and take in protein. Damage to the temporal lobe also means the sense of smell is damaged except that a sense of smell for sweet things, especially sweet baking smells, remains.

As changes in taste and smell become more pronounced, the person with dementia begins to be less interested in food and, as a result, take in fewer calories. This is a problem especially as someone begins to enter the later stages of the disease. One of the behaviors associated with Stage Six (see Chapter 11) is that a person may begin to be in almost constant movement, spending much of her day walking around and around her room or building.

This constant movement burns calories and accelerates weight loss. Unfortunately, this is usually about the same time she begins to exhibit an apparent disinterest in daily nutrition or hydration needs. As this stage progresses, she will begin to suffer from dramatic weight loss and for the first time she will begin to take on the look of dementia with a drawn, withered, lost and disheveled appearance.

Bob's Story

A client once called me to describe a problem with her husband, retired engineer who had been diagnosed with Alzheimer's. With great frustration, she detailed his disinterest in food and his continual walking around their home. When I asked if he had lost weight, she reported he was down at least 30 pounds. When I asked if he was craving sweets, she blurted out "Oh he tries, he tries to eat the pie, but I won't let him!" She really wouldn't let him have any dessert until he ate his other food. Because he wouldn't eat his other food, he never got his sweet rewards.

What the wife didn't understand was that he wanted pie, cake, cookies and ice cream because he could only taste those sweet things. In concern for his health, she wanted to make certain he continued to take in nutrition from the other food groups and was oblivious to the calorie count for his day. No one had explained taste changes to her or how they would impact her husband.

⟶

Once a person begins to be disinterested in regular foods but begins craving sweets, the challenge is to get her to eat. Eventually, interest in food will be lost. No amount of sweetener or coaxing will encourage the person to take in nutrition. But before that time, finding creative ways to make the food more tasty and appealing becomes the challenge for caregivers.

The trick is to disguise the foods. Things such as syrup, barbecue sauce, ketchup, sugar, honey, brown sugar, applesauce and jams are routinely used as sweeteners so that a person with later stage dementia will eat and enjoy the food. (If someone is diabetic, consult with a dietitian for ways to sweeten food.)

It is not unusual to be in a memory community and see applesauce on a pork chop or syrup on eggs as a way to enhance the taste of food and increase a person's caloric intake. Also, baking cookies, muffins and bread can be pleasant for everyone. A daily activity that includes stirring the baking mixture, enjoying the smell while it cooks and eating the cake as a snack can be fun and add calories to the day.

At some point, most families will begin to focus on keeping up total calorie count instead of ensuring a well-balanced diet of proteins, carbohydrates and vegetables. Remember, the disease is terminal. Better nutrition will not slow the progression of the disease.

Persons with dementia also need increased hydration to help their bodies avoid infection. If you or I were to stop drinking fluids today, we might get a headache, but probably would not develop an infection. For an Alzheimer's person, however, failure to take in enough liquids quickly makes her prone especially to a urinary tract infection.

UTI Risk

In many cases, someone who has dementia will not be able to tell you about her UTI. Because of damage in the brain, she may not feel, remember or understand the burning sensation that occurs when she pees is a sign that she has a bladder infection or a urinary tract infection (UTI). Normally, during urination (when you pee), if there is an infection you will feel intense pain in the front or back of the kidneys, or in the bladder.

Your urine may have blood in it, or have strong smell. You may even feel like sharp glass is poking you when you are urinating. These feelings of pain, the sight of blood, etc., alert you to seek medical help. She may or may not feel any pain, remember to tell you about the pain, or recognize her urine is the wrong color or has streaks of blood in it.

To make matters worse, UTIs for someone with dementia and can cause delirium and even death. Always be alert to the possibility of a UTI in your loved one. Once UTIs begin, they will be a constant danger for your loved one.

The deceptive UTI becomes a diagnosis of Chronic UTI and remains a threat. Be alert to sudden changes in behavior over a day or few hours.

These behavioral changes include aggression, agitation, restlessness or lethargy. These are all indicators that something different is happening. The most frequent and common infection is a UTI.

Again, the reason is not a toileting problem; it is not inattention by the caregiving staff. She may be getting plenty of fluids and not be dehydrated at all, but still develop the infection. The UTIs are occurring because of the damage in her brain. They are part of dementia.

Other causes of UTIs may be delirium, medication changes or interactions, constipation, depression, excessive urine output, restricted mobility, vaginitis or atrophic urethritis.

Notify your loved one's physician at once, especially if you see dark, even orange colored, or strong smelling urine. Don't rely on the person with dementia to alert you to the infection!

Because a person with dementia has less interest in hydration or liquids, almost any type of fluid will do. If someone does not enjoy water, give them juice or iced decaffeinated tea. Just be cautious of providing liquids that contain caffeine, as a damaged brain cannot process caffeine.

Eliminating a person's routine drinking substances can be challenging, especially if a person is used to them. In the case of caffeine, don't just stop providing it cold turkey. This will cause a withdrawal headache for your loved one. Instead, take a week or more to slowly wean a person from the caffeine by gradually replacing it with a decaffeinated version of the tea or coffee or dark colored sodas.

Alcohol

The same goes for alcohol, though in many cases the drinking of these sorts of beverages is a lifestyle habit rather than a physical addition. In some instances, caregivers find it better to simply substitute a non-alcoholic drink so that the person with dementia can continue to enjoy the camaraderie of a social happy hour without further damaging her brain. People with advanced dementia usually cannot tell the difference between the regular and numerous alcohol-free versions of wine and beer.

I once knew two gentlemen who had dementia and lived in a memory community in San Antonio. Families of both men reported to the executive director that their fathers enjoyed an afternoon beer and snack. Whenever I visited this community around 3 p.m., I could find these two white-haired men sitting at a table facing the backyard where they share a bowl of pretzels and two icy mugs of non-alcoholic beer every day.

For those with dementia who were also alcoholics, the promise of a cold beer or glass of wine (non-alcoholic, of course) may be the only way to get them to participate in social activities.

Interestingly, persons with dementia who are given non-alcohol beverages often will behave as though they had been drinking real alcohol.

When you are debating whether or not to follow this advice, keep this in mind: alcohol is a neurotoxin. That is, it is technically a poison. Your brain processes alcohol when it is consumed. If your loved one is a Stage Five person, she already has a half-pound of brain tissue gone. Given the fall risks, the brain damage, and the danger of alcohol, the decision to not allow the drink seems fairly easy to make.

Doing so can be considered to be ethically and medically irresponsible. Despite scientific evidence that alcohol and caffeine are harmful to dementia patients, some memory care companies will insist that a person has the right to drink whatever that she wants unless she has a doctor's order. A high-quality, dementia-specific program will understand that a dementia brain is damaged and not serve alcohol.

If you as a caregiver are drinking, be aware the amount of alcohol recommended for adults is now four ounces of red wine daily. It is no longer a "drink," but red wine. To help your brain process alcohol if you are drinking, try sipping water between sips of your drink. The water helps protect your brain as it processes the alcohol.

Thomas' Story

The activity department at a community where I once worked in Virginia decided to throw a carnival party for all five floors of a skilled care facility. The team planned a bingo tournament and raffle, a fishing booth, a cakewalk, and a variety of other games.

Food and drink included hot dogs, hamburgers, cotton candy and popcorn, orange, grape and lime sodas and non-alcoholic beer iced down in several washtubs. At the end of the party we were taking one of the residents back to his room by wheelchair after his fifth "beer."

Normally quite steady and ambulatory, Thomas, a retired Navy veteran, opted for a wheelchair ride back to his room after a long day outside. Suddenly he slid out of the chair to a very surprised sitting position on the ground. As I supported him and waited for the director of nursing to ensure he hadn't hurt himself, Thomas looked up at me, grinned and said, "That party was better than the Navy parties."

He even slurred his words a bit. Professionals in dementia buildings everywhere report this same tipsy behavior among residents whenever they enjoy a non-alcoholic happy hour. The reason is a result of the camaraderie of the party rather than alcohol and a bit of learned behavior that tells you if you've been drinking at a party, you must be a bit tipsy.

Coping with changing taste perceptions and the need to eliminate certain beverages can be dealt with by using the following tips:

- Take advantage of a person's remaining taste for sweets to keep her caloric intake high. Provide additional sweet snacks, including candy, throughout the day to supplement the calorie count and make adjustments with your physician if your loved one is diabetic. If someone wants to start with dessert or only eat dessert, pick your battle. Start the meal with dessert then try introducing a sandwich or smaller meal again in a half hour or so.

- To increase liquid intake, provide plenty of tempting sweet options, such as sweet tea, chocolate or strawberry-flavored milk, apple juice and prune juice, and milk shakes.

- Always praise your loved one for eating, chewing and swallowing. Positive reinforcement helps with any dementia activity, including those that take place at mealtime.

- If mom continues to demand morning coffee or an evening glass of wine or scotch, keep in mind that what likely is at work is not the need for either but a craving for familiarity and old habits. Again, don't fight the battle. Instead, put decaffeinated coffee in a favorite mug or pour sparkling grape juice into fancy wine glass. Chances are the person with dementia will not know the difference, especially as the disease progresses.

Interpreting Sound

People in general tend to have some level of hearing loss as they age because of normal age-related structural changes in the ear. In addition to normal aging changes, some persons have additional medical conditions that cause hearing impairments.

Veterans may have sustained damage during their service due to explosions or artillery fire. Others may have hearing loss from an accident or illness.

Those with Alzheimer's, however, face additional problems as their temporal lobes (hearing, language and smell) fall prey to the disease. In the case of dementia, the brain is unable to translate noise it hears or determine the direction from which a sound originates. Complicating these changes in hearing perception are the effects of aphasia, the inability to use or understand language, along with amnesia, the inability to use short- or long-term memory.

Although hearing aids for Alzheimer's persons can be helpful, they usually come with additional problems. First, memory loss means they may not remember to wear their hearing aids. They also may not remember or understand how to adjust a hearing aid or recognize when the batteries need replacing.

And as the person enters the later stages of the dementia process, hearing aids, along with eyeglasses and dentures, are likely to get tossed in the trash. Items such as hearing aids often end up in the trash because a person with dementia suffers from an inability to recognize or use common objects (agnosia and amnesia). When a person suddenly discovers an object in her ear and doesn't recognize it or understand its purpose, chances are it will be tossed away.

The same concept applies to eyeglasses and dentures or jewelry. Instead of getting angry at your loved one or blaming her or other caregivers for throwing away expensive items such as these, make it a habit to use trashcans with tight lids. And always check the trash, especially the ones near someone's bedside or in the bathroom, before disposing of the contents.

Keep in mind the following tips:

- Eliminate unnecessary distracting sounds, such as the television or radio.
- Use a lower pitch of voice when speaking to someone with advanced dementia. The brain will hear this tone better and give the individual a better chance of translating the sounds.
- When speaking to someone, face her so she can see your face.
- Speak slowly, clearly and calmly. Shouting at a person can be misinterpreted as anger and can cause an outburst. Chewing food or gum while speaking to someone makes your words even more difficult to understand and may be interpreted as rude.

Interpreting Touch, Temperature and Pain

The sense of touch remains strong throughout life, even for Alzheimer's people who have lost their abilities to translate what they see, hear, smell and taste. This means you have the opportunity to provide a tactile environment that both stimulates and calms your loved one.

In the later stages of the disease, you may notice repetitive hand movements. Common behaviors include folding napkins, taking tissues out of a box and folding them, or tearing rolls of toilet paper apart square by square and folding each piece. It is not unusual for families to discover drawers full of nothing but neatly folded tissue or paper.

Another common repetitive hand movement seen in a dementia person is the rubbing together of her fingertips (pilling) or rubbing her fingertips on her thighs when sitting. All of these are normal behaviors. The only time you really need to be concerned is if someone starts picking or scratching her skin in a way that causes wounds.

The reason behind these actions include the following: 1) Most dementia people today are from a generation of people who did not sit idle and stare into space. Most people get bored easily with nothing to do. 2) People have an inherent need to be needed and to be helpful. (Examples to try are located below in this chapter).

The ability of the brain to translate information that relates to temperature also is compromised in the dementia person. In normal aging, our bodies cool slightly as circulation slows and skin thins. We also engage in less intense activities.

An 80-year-old person simply doesn't move as much as 60-, 40- or a 4-year-old. Generally, the body core temperature of an Alzheimer's patient is just a bit lower than her non-dementia peers. This normally would not be a problem except that the damaged brain cannot tell circulation to increase to compensate for the lower temperature. This is why memory communities are warmer than what is comfortable for most people. The building's temperature is set for the person with dementia, not the staff.

Pat's Story

If you have ever been in Washington D.C. during August, you experienced its hot, humid and uncomfortable weather. In one climate-controlled building, I met a lady who complained of being cold despite wearing a t-shirt, turtleneck, sweater, muffler, gloves, pants, socks and hat. Pat would walk unsteadily down the hallway, complaining of being cold, even while wearing all her clothing.

Following one particularly nasty fall, Pat was sent to the emergency room as a precaution. The CAT scan of her head was performed. The results clearly showed deterioration in her parietal lobes, which explained her need to be dressed warmly. In Pat's brain and body, she really was cold.

People With Dementia Are Cold

Because many Alzheimer's patients don't know if they are too cold or too hot, are unable to verbalize the need to put on or take off a sweater, and are unable to remember how to physically use a sweater or even find one in the first place, a caregiver must be more proactive about ensuring a dementia person is dressed correctly.

The rule of thumb is this: If you need just a shirt, your mom may need a shirt and a t-shirt. If you need a shirt and a t-shirt, she may need a shirt, t-shirt and sweater. Also feel your loved one's hands and feet. If her hands and feet are cold, she is cold and needs more clothing.

Moreover, people who have dementia also can extremely sensitive to pain. The invigorating spray of water from the shower may be perceived by the Alzheimer's brain as a stinging sensation. A belt holding pants up may cause a pinching feeling, so always check it. Tape on an adult diaper may catch and pull at the skin. Keep in mind that expressions of pain from an individual with dementia are not being fabricated on purpose. In her mind, the pain is very real.

Because you know your loved one's brain is damaged and you understand she is having difficulty with language, you may worry that you won't be able to recognize her pain and need for help. Keep in mind that experts report an estimated 70 percent of communication between humans takes place without speech and that you already understand much of it.

Think back to when you were a new parent and cared for an infant who couldn't speak, write or tap out Morse code for assistance. Chances are that within a few days you learned the difference between cries that meant hunger, teeth pain, fever, a need to be held or have a diaper changed, or a reaction to a big brother's pinch. You'll quickly develop these same skills to care for and communicate with someone who has Alzheimer's.

Of course, you will want to ask your loved one if she is in pain when you suspect this may be the case. For example, you walk into the bathroom just in time to see her slip and fall. In the early stages of the disease, you will probably get a good answer. If she says she's okay, she probably is fine.

As the disease progresses, though, you may find she answers differently each time she is asked the same question.

Remember that the right temporal lobe controls singing, cursing and automatic "yes" and "no" responses that are deeply imbedded. About the age of two, we discovered these two words had a great deal of power and that adults around us got excited when we used them. Answering, "yes" to a question ("Yes, I ate all my peas.") usually got us praise while a "no" ("No, I did not pick up my toys.") usually elicited a negative response.

Because this side of the brain tends to function longer in a person with dementia, asking questions of someone in the later stages of the disease does not mean you'll get a correct answer. In many cases, you'll simply get an automatic response without any meaning behind it.

Clues to Pain

When a fall or other accident happens, you'll want to look for clues the same way you would with a young child. Facial indicators (furrowed brows, frowning, wincing); movement changes (sharp and shorter breaths, muscle or body tenseness, pacing, physical agitation, aggression, trembling); vocalizations (moaning, crying, voice pitch changes, cursing, verbal aggression); changes in body position (curling up in a fetal position or kicking out, moving about or laying still, protecting an area on the body from touch or movement); and personality, mood and behavior changes (aggression, combativeness) can all signify someone is feeling differently or is in pain or hurting.

⟜

Here are some additional ideas about how you can provide a varied, appropriate tactile environment:

- Petting an animal is often pleasurable and calming. However, if you fear a person might grab a pet too hard or get scratched or bitten, provide a soft pillow or stuffed animal that uses real fur. Another idea I've seen work well is when the arms of an old rabbit coat purchased at the thrift store are cut off and stuffed with foam and sewn shut. (Touching fur is a very soothing activity for humans, whether they have dementia or not. A pet may even help you stay calm as a caregiver.)

- Providing a basket of socks or washcloths to sort is a safe pastime that addresses the need to repeat motion and movement as well as one's need to feel helpful. Use different textures, and keep colors to dark and white ones so the pieces of material are easier to distinguish from one another. And remember getting your loved one to match the socks is not the goal. Instead, the goal is to provide to an activity she can perform with her hands.

- Provide one or more pots of herbs for to her to water. If she touches the plants, the smells are pleasant. If she tears off a leaf and eats it, the plant is not poisonous.

- In extreme cases of restlessness, talk to a doctor about medications that may help.

Eliminating Stimuli Overload

People with Alzheimer's may become overwhelmed when faced with too many visual and auditory stimuli. Remember, the problem is not that they don't sense what's going on around them; the problem is with how the brain processes and translates what is being seen and heard. A healthy brain applies value to the stimuli input it receives and then determines where it should focus.

Your brain filters noise and movement it deems unnecessary, allowing you to focus on what is most important at that particular time. For most people, multitasking capabilities mean they can process about five or six items at a time. This allows you to talk on the phone while ignoring the television and your spouse talking to a neighbor at the front door all while continuing to make dinner and correct a child who is trying to feed the dog ice cream.

Remember for a person with dementia, the brain slowly loses this filtering system. Too much environmental stimulation (i.e., noise, light, movement and other things we may not even recognize because of our healthy brain's ability to filter the extra stuff) can turn a once-enjoyed activity into a frightening experience for someone with dementia.

Take the process of dining, for example. Too many distractions – music, television, loud talking, movement by others, multiple pieces of glassware and silverware, table decorations, bottles of condiments, even the color of the plate – can be overwhelming to a person with Alzheimer's. Even if your mom always loved going out to dinner, her dementia may advance to a point where she can't go to a restaurant anymore because of the overwhelming noise and activity. She may become frightened, agitated or aggressive instead.

Here are some ideas to help someone deal with information overload

- If your loved one is living in a dementia facility, visit during mealtimes and observe if the staff is taking steps to reduce stimuli during meals. For example, no television or music, but quiet. If your loved one is living at home, keep plates simple and place settings to a bare minimum. Again, turn off the television or radio. If others are at the table, keep conversations quiet and calm. Her brain needs all its ability to focus on eating.

- Minimize distractions in rooms by keeping clutter to a minimum and noises muted. If trying to communicate with a person who has dementia, turn off the television and radio, and move away from others. (More communication techniques are in Chapter 8.)

Now that you better understand the many changes taking place in the environment of an Alzheimer's person because of damage to her brain, you will be able to appreciate how easy it is for that individual to become paranoid, frustrated and angry. Imagine how frightened you would feel if you were being startled and scared by people throughout the day who seemingly jump out at you.

Imagine not understanding what someone says to you or not being able to communicate that your throat is dry and you need a drink of water. Imagine not being able to determine whether a noise you hear is beautiful music or the sound of danger. Imagine not understanding why you are being forced to eat something that tastes like cardboard or being punished for trying to eat the pie (Remember "Oh he tries to eat the pie!").

For these reasons and all we know about the dementia process, it is incumbent on us to do everything possible to make the world of the person we love easier to navigate and understand.

Five Points To Remember

1. **Severe changes in hearing, sight and other sensory perception are more a consequence of damage to the brain from dementia rather than old age.**

2. **Although communication capabilities may be compromised by the Four A's, you can use non-verbal**

communication skills to help decode a dementia person's needs.

3. Visual changes, including a loss peripheral vision and depth perception, can be frightening to a dementia person and cause her to have trouble navigating in a once-familiar environment.

4. Because of changes in taste and smell perception, getting a dementia person to take in enough calories becomes more challenging.

5. You can sooth and engage a dementia person by finding ways to keep her hands busy.

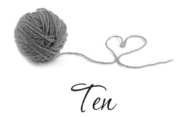

Ten

COMMUNICATION TECHNIQUES

Trying to communicate with someone who has Alzheimer's can become increasingly frustrating as the disease systematically destroys the brain's lobes. Difficulties that begin with your loved one's inability to find the right word evolve into problems understanding what many words or sounds mean.

As she gradually loses her ability to have a train of thought, pay attention or the capacity to follow instructions, the combination of background noise, hearing changes and sensitivity to tone and body language may make a normal conversation very challenging. In many cases, your attempts at conversation may actually cause her to become agitated.

In spite of these challenges, you should not give up on communication. If you are the primary caregiver, you want to ensure your loved one's daily needs are being met physically and socially. If your loved one has moved to a memory care community or a skilled care facility, you will want to find a way to make your visits meaningful to both of you.

And although your ability to communicate with your loved one will never return to the way it was before dementia struck, the following tips will help make communication easier and less frustrating.

Visit Preparation

Visits by friends and family members will be better for everyone if they know what to expect. Depending upon where in the dementia process your loved one is and how long it has been since the visitor has seen her, he or she may be shocked at the changes that have taken place. On the other hand, they may wonder if anything is even wrong.

Don't forget that physical symptoms of dementia often don't reveal themselves until the later stages of the disease. Add in the fact that automatic social conversation responses often remain strong long after other skills have been lost, and visitors may actually miss cognition challenges.

Be careful to not allow yourself or others be fooled into thinking that your loved one has rebounded or is getting better, or has given a correct "yes" or "no" answer to a question. It is not unusual however, to see a change and increase in ability when a socially isolated person is placed in a community. The increased activity and interactions with others can boost your loved one's responses for a time.

Finally, don't plan long visits, as people with dementia tire quickly. Limit visits from 15 minutes to an hour. It is common to believe only you can provide proper care for your loved one. And in many ways, that is probably true, after all, you know her best.

But communities have a fresh caregiver there every eight hours. These are trained professionals who don't carry guilt or remorse or feelings of anger or frustration with them as they provide care.

For the most part, our professional care partners are talented and dedicated people, doing incredible jobs providing for our frailest adults. Trust them to do their jobs.

Approach

There is a proper way to approach a person with dementia. Because her ability to understand the world around her is impaired, approaching from the front is key. This allows the person a chance to translate that someone is moving towards them, it gives a damaged brain an opportunity to translate movement and determine who the person approaching is.

The approach from the front must be slower than normal movement. It is a slower way of moving on your part, but the benefits are well worth it. Practice your approach at one step per second. Again, you are allowing the person with dementia's brain time to translate the movement and motion forward.

The caregiver needs to approach and stop in the normal distance between people. Avoid leaning over the person, as this move can be perceived as threatening. Once you have reached your loved one, you should move to the best side of the person with dementia. In other words, if the person has had a stroke and is left side impaired, then the caregiver should move to the strong side or her right side.

Once on the person's side, the care partner should introduce herself, shake hands and greet the person and kneel down. Just because someone has dementia, it doesn't give us the right to forget our manners.

Now reality is that most of us are not able to kneel down and pop back up, especially over and over throughout the day. Instead keep a chair on the side of your person so that you can sit down next to her. Or step back and bend over, again the point is to be below her and not over the top of her.

Facing the person from the front is known as "Confrontational Stance." Facing the person from the side is called the "Supportive Stance." The Supportive Stance gives the person with dementia the perception of control, in that she can turn away from the caregiver, rather than feeling trapped or fearful.

This may feel silly at first, but you have to remember this: A person with dementia is operating with a diminished brain, while you are not.

The correct approach and movement to the side is less frightening to her. Sitting on the side of her, rather than leaning over the top of her gives her the impression that she is in control. It makes her feel safer. And if you are annoying her, she can simply turn away.

If the caregiver leaves for even a few seconds, this approach should be used again as the person with dementia may not remember the caregiver was just there and stepped away for a moment.

I realize this approach sounds tiring, but remember, your loved one's world is making less and less sense to her. It is incumbent upon us to make her feel as safe as possible.

"No, No, No!"

Leaning over a person is simply not done. It is confusing and if the dementia person is a fight person, then the caregiver may get struck. If the dementia person is a flight person, then she may get hurt trying to get away from the caregiver. If the dementia person is a freeze person, then she is being frightened by poor caregiving.

Approaching a dementia person from behind is not done for the same reasons. The person may not hear your approach and you may frighten or startle her and again you may get struck. But the key point is that you may frighten her. Your face upside down or at a funny angle is even harder for her brain to figure out.

So remember this: approach her from the front. Go slow at about one second per step. When you reach her, introduce yourself and move to her side. Make yourself lower than she is, either by kneeling down or by sitting in a chair or bending and stepping back. Get low. This is the approach you should use every time.

Communication

We covered some communication skills in Chapters Five, Six and Seven. It is important to recognize that the person with dementia may or may not be able to understand speech. Remember automatic "yes/no" responses remain until speech is lost. When your loved one answers "yes" or "no" it does not mean she understands what "yes" or "no" actually mean.

When you need to or just want to sit and visit with your loved one, get prepared. This means you will turn off the television, radio, music, etc. Her brain needs to be able to focus on the conversation and since she may have reached the stage where she cannot filter out background noise, you have to be more aware.

It is also important that you know the person's history. If you work with this generation, you should know their history and culture. That means who the presidents were, the wars, aspects of the war like a Victory Garden, ration stamps, Axis powers, Allied powers, etc. You should know songs and movies and popular sayings. Know the person's family, children, spouse, parents, grandparents, etc. Learn her birthplace, family background, favorite foods, colors, hobbies and job experience.

These things are important. Since she is using old files to converse, you have to have an understanding of who she is and where she is from. Be prepared to take your time, speak in short sentences, and repeat information, repeat information, repeat information.

Another "No, No, No!"

Do not quiz the person with dementia. Questions should not be used in conversation. This is a tricky technique to learn but think about this. Isn't it uncomfortable to be asked "Do you know who I am?" or "Who is this person?" especially when you don't?

Remember, she may not recognize anyone either. We don't enjoy persons approaching us that way and neither do persons with dementia. It is embarrassing and persons with dementia can feel embarrassment.

As the disease progresses, try giving her information when you greet her. Instead of the "Do you know who

I am?', try "Hi, I am Jimmie, your only son. I am better looking than your other children, Brenda and Ronnie. I was always smarter and you always liked me more." This approach has used humor, named off other family members and given the person with dementia information she may be able to grasp. Make sure to train visiting friends and family members to do the same.

Her brain is being destroyed, this is not "use it or lose it." To question persons with dementia is considered rude and cruel. People with dementia are doing the best they can.

By Stage Five of the disease process, it is thought the person with dementia is able to understand three out of four words. By the end of the disease, she will understand no words, but she can still understand tone. Balance her decline with the knowledge that this is still an adult and she should not be talked to as though she is a child.

In the end, sometimes the only communication skill needed is to sit quietly and hold your loved one's hand.

Environment

As discussed earlier, people with dementia can become easily distracted or overwhelmed by too much stimuli. This can make already challenging conversations more difficult. For this reason, you'll want to ensure the surroundings in which you have a conversation are the best possible for your loved one.

The person with dementia's brain needs to be able to focus on the conversation. Remember she cannot filter out background noise, and you may need to supply information to jump start her brain.

One important thing you can do is to eliminate noise distractions, such as televisions and radios. If possible, simply turn them off or turn down the volume. You'll also want to get away from the conversations of others. If you are visiting a community and find your loved one in a group setting, move to a quiet area without other residents.

In addition to eliminating distractions, you will avoid drawing the attention of other people who have dementia and want to be a part of your conversation. Don't be alarmed if this happens, however. A person with advanced dementia has lost some inhibition and impulse control, so joining up with your group doesn't seem abnormal to her. If the "visitor" is disruptive, just ask the staff to distract her with another activity.

Because the vision and hearing of a dementia patient is likely diminished, do what you can to make it easier for her to see and hear you. Encourage her to use her glasses and hearing aids.

Also ensure you are in an area with good lighting, sit about an arm's length away at eye level and ensure that your face can be seen when you are speaking. Lean forward to increase volume but do not give the appearance of shouting as this can be misinterpreted as anger. Do not have chewing gum or candy in your mouth, and do not cover your mouth while you are talking.

Conversation Clues

I cannot stress enough that one of the worst things you or someone else can do to a loved one who has dementia is to ask "Do you remember me?" or "Who am I?" This is just as embarrassing for her as it would be for you if a person you should recognize, but don't, asked you that question. You must remember her brain is being destroyed and so this is not "use it or lose it" situation.

This is not a teaching moment and this is not a way to help someone with dementia. To ask questions like this to people with dementia is rude and cruel. People with dementia are doing the best they can. Being quizzed wasn't fun in grade school and isn't not fun as an adult.

One key to holding successful conversations with people who suffer from dementia is to supply them with information that will allow them to participate. If it is hot outside and your family always went to the beach in the summer, discuss those memories. During November for example, talk about special family foods associated with Thanksgiving. Hints such as these allow an individual's social skills and possibly old memories to take over so that she can add to the conversation.

Here Are Examples:

- "Hi, Dillon. I am Billy. I was your neighbor when you and your wife Erin lived at the beach. Your son Jackson was a toddler then. He played with my kids Denver and Davyn in the ocean and they built sand castles."
- "Hi, MeMa. I'm your favorite granddaughter Kyla. I was thinking about my wedding to Tanner and how you made your famous pound cakes for our rehearsal dinner."

These approaches use social skills, humor, name other family members and give the person with dementia information or clues she may be able to grasp.

If you don't share memories with the individual or the memories you have are too recent for her to recall, you'll find it helpful to know that person's personal history (i.e., parent names, birthplace, favorite foods and activities, employment history) as well as her generation's history (i.e., presidents, wars, popular songs and sayings, dances) and use those memories to enjoy a conversation. Remember Loraine's missing pants were solved because the clue "army" pants meant World War II military uniforms and khaki!

Use a person's name frequently, but do not use pet names or terms of endearment (i.e., "sweetie" or "honey") unless you know the person well and used those names prior to dementia. And a person with Alzheimer's should never be called "Grandma" or "my girlfriend" or something similar by a visitor or caregiver unless she actually is that person's grandmother or girlfriend.

Who Are You Talking To?

People with dementia may not remember their spouses; it depends upon the stage of dementia they are in. Think about the filing cabinet. This means a woman may not respond to her married name. In other words, Mrs. Smith may not remember Mr. Smith and, therefore, only remembers her maiden name. When she reaches this stage, calling Mrs. Smith by her first name will be less confusing to her.

Think about Judy's mother and her confusion over how Judy could possibly be her daughter. When you are in a community and staff members are addressing ladies by their first name, they are not being rude. They are doing so because those ladies remember their first names and not their married names.

As the disease progresses, the ability of someone with dementia to understand abstract thoughts and concepts, and the ability to answer questions becomes more difficult. So avoid asking open-ended questions such as "What did you have for breakfast?" unless you supply the answers.

Instead, try something more like this: "Hi, Mom. I'm your daughter Kayli. Did you have breakfast today? It looks like you've had a good breakfast with eggs and pancakes and bacon. I know you love bacon."

Asking a question this way gives your mom hints she needs to answer and join the conversation.

Pace and Tone

Because a person with dementia has challenges processing information, speech and language, you must recognize that the person with dementia may or may not be able to understand what you are trying to communicate. In the beginning of the disease process, it is thought the person with dementia is able to understand three out of four words.

By the end stage, she will not understand words at all, though she will comprehend tone of voice. Regardless of the dementia stage, break your conversations into smaller units for greater clarity and understanding. If you use short sentences instead of long, rambling sentences, your loved one's brain has a better chance of processing information. And pause frequently and check for comprehension.

Valerie's Story

*L*et me stress conversation skills with a story. Valerie was a retired Army officer. She married another military intelligence officer and was one of the first female officers to arrive in Japan at the war's end. She had a thousand stories of the war and was just a delightful lady.

She was also the daughter of a diplomat who served in Europe prior to World War II. In talking with Valerie one day I asked if she and her brothers enjoyed going up over seas.

"Yes, yes we loved it," she replied. As our conversation continued I asked if she enjoyed skiing and ice skating while in Europe and again she replied, "Yes, yes, we loved it."

Eventually I asked if her mother was a good cook. "Crook!" Valerie suddenly shouted. "Crook! My mother was no crook!" Our conversation took a nosedive.

*Remember, it is very important to speak clearly.

Also keep in mind the brain's capacity to translate sound correctly is impaired. This impacts one's ability to determine the source of sound and recognize people's voices. Lower pitches are picked up more readily than higher pitches, so women should try to lower the pitch of their voices.

You are communicating with an adult, so never talk to someone as though she were a child. This means you should eliminate baby talk or a patronizing tone of voice. Instead, try to use a tone similar to how you spoke to your children, soft and loving with gentle touches. You also will want to avoid speaking with an exaggeratedly slow rate, a higher pitch, exaggerated intonation or shouting.

One time when pace and tone are especially helpful is when you want your loved one to follow directions. Depending upon the stage of the disease, simple and clear instructions are most helpful. Break each task into its smaller components and, with a clear and calm voice, describe what you are doing for and with someone at each step.

Also give praise and encouragement at each step. For example, dressing an adult with Stage Five dementia would go something like this: "Good morning, Joe. It is a beautiful morning outside, but a little cold. Let's get your blue sweater to put on. I'll help you. Put your right arm out first. Good. Now let's put the right sleeve on. Good, you are doing great. Let's bring the sweater around. Good. Now let's put your left hand through the sleeve. Good. You are doing so well. Soon we'll have this sweater on. Okay, that was wonderful. You always look so good in your blue sweater."

If you observe professional caregivers such as certified nursing assistants and nurses, the best ones always use the short sentence and lots of praise when communicating. The top ones will provide at least 10 positive responses for each dressing activity. This can be tiring, but it works. Remember, people tend to believe anyone can provide care to a person with dementia. But in reality, care for dementia is more complex, challenging and difficult because of what the disease is doing to your loved one's brain.

Non-Verbal Communication

As your loved one begins to lose her language skills, you'll need to pay more attention to her non-verbal communication. Look closely at how she holds her body, and watch her facial expressions for clues about what she is trying to communicate. You'll also want to be aware of your own body language. Avoid signs of impatience and annoyance, as these are noticeable even to a person with dementia and can impede communication.

If you do run into conversation roadblocks, try incorporating gestures, pantomime and pointing as a supplement to words. You might even have success with a communication book or board. A small eraser board – white with black markers only please – may work for a person with hearing impairment. Use simple words and watch to make certain she is following the conversation.

Just as importantly, don't be afraid to touch someone who has dementia. Shaking hands is another way to communicate, especially for this generation of elderly. A simple handshake allows for a quick and positive interaction. Shaking hands also allows you to redirect your loved one away from others or distract her if she is becoming combative. Remember to shake hands properly however, or this will result in more problems. A firm handshake and direct eye contact are critical.

Even when words fail, you will be able to convey affection and reassurance through simple gestures of touch. You might want to bring lotion and offer a hand, arm, leg or foot massage. Touching will be therapeutic for both of you, and the lotion will help her dry skin.

When you are sitting with your loved one and talking, feel free to hold her hand or touch her arm. Sitting quietly and holding hands may be the final activity for some families. Slight pressure on the palm is also soothing for many persons with dementia.

Develop a Communication Book

A communication book is a photo album with pictures and words of common objects your loved might need, such as a glass for thirsty, a sandwich for hungry or a toilet for bathroom needs.

If your loved one speaks a language that you don't or if she lives in a community where no one else speaks her language, be certain to take along her book. The staff needs to know how to say things that range from "hello" or "good night" to "bathroom" or "hungry."

Write the word in large letters for your mom, phonetically for the staff and include a picture of the item if possible.

Multilingual Challenges

As mentioned in an earlier chapter, persons who are bilingual will gradually lose their second language. Because memory is being removed in a reverse order, the language that has been learned longest is retained longest. So if a woman with Alzheimer's was raised speaking Spanish and learned English as a second language, she will eventually remember only the Spanish.

If a person was raised in an English-speaking family but moved to Europe and learned additional languages, she will forget those languages and remember only English as the disease progresses. This can be very challenging to children who never learned a parent's first language or to professional caregivers who work with residents who came from diverse countries.

Eventually, families and caretakers will have to rely on signs and communication books in the individual's native language to communicate.

Show Your Manners

As mentioned throughout this book, the generation most likely to suffer from dementia today has deeply embedded social skills. So just because someone is unable to carry on a normal conversation does not mean she will not recognize disrespectful or derogatory comments, or feel isolated or insulted if others speak about her as if she were not in the room. Even if someone is unresponsive, you have no idea what she actually hears or understands.

This means you must always assume that your loved one is aware of what is going on around her and adjust your conversations appropriately when she is nearby. Doctors, nurses or anyone else in her area should always let her know they are talking about her and ask permission to do so. Your loved one deserves the same common courtesies we all expect.

Also take care not to embarrass people with dementia. This chapter already discussed why you should not ask an

Alzheimer's person if she remembers you. Another thing you should not ask is why she did or did not do something. Answering these sorts of questions requires a higher level of brain functioning that is not possible in those with dementia, so she likely will not be able to answer.

If you need to get information, rewording the question and providing conversation clues may help. This same inability to use higher brain functioning also means people with dementia don't respond well to arguments. Because she is unable to make her point and unable to understand your reasoning, your attempts to reason and explain will just cause frustration for both of you and may trigger her to react negatively.

Finally, always remember to maintain the social roles of conversation. Encourage your loved one to talk and listen to what she says – even when it no longer makes sense. When it comes to this point, respond to the tone of the conversation. If she is laughing, then laugh with her. If she seems to be upset, pat her hand reassuringly and tell her all will be okay.

You have this skill and use it all the time with other people. You may meet someone and suddenly realize you haven't been paying attention to the conversation, so you respond to the facial expressions. This is the same thing.

No doubt communication with a loved one who has dementia can be excruciatingly frustrating. Keep in mind, though, a time will come when your mom, dad, spouse, brother, sister, son, daughter or grandparent will no longer be able to have a conversation and you'll remember these times fondly.

Izora's Story

I have to share an Izora story with you.

Izora was a diminutive little lady originally from North Carolina. I loved her dearly. She was quite feisty, at times threatening the caregiving staff with her "walking stick" for taking too long to make her bed or for being strangers in her "house."

She had a daughter that loved her dearly and three times a week Lucy boarded three different buses to make the trek from her apartment to the dementia community.

Now sometimes, as a person works backwards through her files, she will remember an old habit and believe it is a current habit. Izora remembered she enjoyed an occasional cigarette.

Keep in mind Lucy wasn't aware her mother had ever smoked, the smoking habit had happened before Lucy was born.

On the day of the carnival, Lucy arrived to find her mother sitting happily under the pavilion. Izora had a stuffed animal on her lap she won throwing a dart at the balloon board. She had a box of popcorn and a hot dog at the table, a cold "beer" in one hand and a lit cigarette in the other.

"Momma," Lucy cried. "You don't smoke! Now put that cigarette out!"

Izora looked up at her daughter and slowly got out of her chair, all 4'8" tall, she fixed her much larger daughter with an icy stare.

"Child," she growled, "you better remember this. I brought you in this world and I can still take you out!"

Note: Izora finished her cigarette, ate her hotdog and drank her "beer." As I walked by, she looked up and said, "This is the best party ever!" The smoke cleared, her daughter enjoyed the rest of the day, a few months later Izora forgot she had ever smoked.

Five Points To Remember

1. **Do not embarrass someone by asking her questions she is unable to answer. In other words, don't quiz your loved one and don't allow others to quiz her!**

2. **Use common memories and some-one's personal history to jumpstart conversations.**

3. Ensure that possible distractions are minimized when trying to communicate.

4. Be careful about how you approach a person so that she is not startled or frightened.

5. Use touch and tone of voice to communicate when spoken communication is impossible.

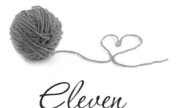

Eleven

ADLs AND CHALLENGING BEHAVIORS

It may seem odd I am putting the Activities of Daily Living (ADLs) and challenging behaviors together, but bear with me.

The ADLs are those things you and I do each day, throughout the day, some of them multiple times, that allow us to function safely in our homes. They are the steps you took this morning and are easy to remember this way.

I woke up (sleeping). I walked to the bathroom (ambulation). I used the bathroom (toileting). I brushed my teeth and combed my hair (grooming). I showered (bathing). I put on clothes (dressing). I had breakfast (eating).

A person with dementia is losing the ability to perform these ADLs herself. She can't remember the steps or interpret signals from her body. She can't figure out how the bathtub works, remember that she needs to shower, know how to find her shoes or put them on properly.

Because of dementia, she may not understand the need to perform these ADLs, some of them the basic physical needs of all humans. As a result, most of the challenging behaviors caregivers face revolve around trying to help.

Please note dementias that attack the frontal lobes will probably be more challenging. These behaviors may only be able to be controlled with medications. It is not uncommon a person with extreme behaviors will need to be evaluated at a geriatric psychiatric hospital for two or more weeks.

This placement in a "geri-psych" means medical professionals who specialize in aging and dementia will examine your loved one. She may need to have medications evaluated and adjusted, for her safety and for the safety of those around her.

Being evaluated in the hospital is nothing to be embarrassed about. What if your loved one had cancer? Would you deny her the chance to be properly treated? Of course not. Medical treatment for behaviors caused by dementia is no different.

Care Giving Tips for Challenging Behaviors

Most care giving challenges occur during the morning simply because that's when most of the daily care giving occurs. The bulk of the ADLs happen when we first wake up. The second most common time for disruptive behavior is the evening, when again, ADLs need to be completed to prepare for bed. And then any meal or incontinent episode can cause a person with dementia to become upset.

These are the tips for completing each of these tasks. In them you may find the combination that works best for your loved one. If you do, take note. You will need to share this information with other caregivers, both assisting in your home or in dementia communities.

When you are assisting with ADLs, put your loved one's hand over your hand and guide her through the steps of the task. This will help clue her brain for a bit longer. She will be less likely to resist care because her brain will recognize the movement, but not necessarily your hand. This is the "hand over hand" technique used by professionals.

Sleeping: Throughout the day, raise the blinds, turn on the lights and open the curtains, keep the house bright, This will help to keep your loved one awake and active during the day (but remember in the final stage she will sleep more and more). Rather than order her to bed, stretch, yawn and tell her you are ready for bed. Help her put on her pajamas.

Before bed, ensure her bladder is empty, and calmly orient her to surroundings if need be. Reassure her that you are there. If needed, provide a small cup of warm milk as a mild sleep aid. (Eliminate caffeine from her diet entirely.) Provide nighttime lighting and simplify the bedding and furnishings, to keep her safe if she needs the bathroom. During the day, if possible only allow her to nap in living room -- not bedroom. Napping in the bedroom adds to her confusion about day and night. And excessive napping interferes with nighttime sleep.

Ambulation: At times, she may simply not be able to remember how to walk from one part of the day to the next. Always eliminate medical causes, making certain she hasn't been hurt from a fall or fractured a bone. Simplify her environment, eliminate clutter, use non-skid mats or no mats or rugs, check her shoes for comfort, and help her to use good body mechanics. Remember to use night-lights, limit rearranging furniture or arrange furniture to allow her to use it as support, install railings, and protect her from stairways, possibly by closing the opening with a locked door.

Toileting: Again, you as the caregiver must eliminate medical causes. That is make certain she is not suffering from a UTI or other infection. Help her establish regular routines. Does she go to the bathroom for her bowels in the morning or evening, once a day or once every two days. Does she have loose stools or is she constipated? Watch and observe her for non-verbal cues, such as wiggling, holding herself or agitation. Increase her fluid intake during the day and restrict fluids just before bedtime. Keep her dressed in manageable clothing as this makes going to the bathroom easier. Use incontinence aids (diapers), and make signs or photos to alert her to the location of the bathroom.

Keep the "90-second-rule" in mind. This rule says 90 seconds after eating or drinking, persons with dementia will need a bathroom. It is just a general rule. If something goes in the body, something must come out. It is how we learned to toilet as toddlers and it makes sense. It is also much easier to clean a person who used the toilet, than to have to clean a person with a soiled diaper.

Hygiene: Help her maintain her lifelong routine. If she showered in the morning, allow her to shower in the morning. Simplify the task and environment as much as possible. This can mean putting away all the extra stuff in the bathroom as it can just confuse her more. Use lotion to keep her skin supple and follow good oral hygiene techniques. Baby toothpaste may be easier for her to use as it is sweet. Adult toothpaste may make her mouth feel like it is burning.

Bathing: Maintain her past bathing routine and prepare the bathroom in advance. Remember to keep the bathroom warm, comfortable and inviting. Provide for her safety in the tub or shower, using railings or a chair and handheld shower. Use a soapy sponge or washcloth to distract her if she is modest.

You might try singing with her or talking during the task to divert her attention and her embarrassment. Check temperature of the water, gently coach and praise at each step, use a soapy washcloth or sponge for her to hold and help. And it is okay to se a bribe like a piece of candy. Remember the object of bathing is to clean skin, not dunk a person in water or terrify her. Dry her skin well and check her for injuries and irritation (pink skin in skin/bone spots).

If the shower hurts, try turning the pressure down. You also can protect any skin area by covering the skin with a towel to stop the water from directly hitting it. Always start a shower from the feet and move up. It is less frightening for the person being showered.

Dressing and Grooming: Lay out her clothes in the order they go on. To help her as the disease progresses, reduce the amount of clothes in her closets and drawers. Look for items with elastic waistbands, Velcro tape, tube socks and slip-on shoes, to help her. Keep her warm and comfortable. As the disease advances, move her to loose fitting clothes, but keep her well groomed. She may require a shorter haircut than in the past. She may look disheveled immediately following getting dressed; this is a late stage feature of dementia. Keep her nails manicured, toes too! Try bright colors as a change up. Remember to see the dentist, as tooth decay is dangerous for people with dementia. The infection is very close to the brain, plus broken teeth can add to rapid weight loss.

Nutrition (Eating) and Mealtimes: Maintain her regular eating routine, serving balanced meals and familiar foods. You may need to use diet supplements, secure forbidden foods (diabetics forget they can't have sweets) and serve foods and liquids at a lukewarm temperature. In time you will need to cut her food into small pieces. As the disease progresses, you might serve one food at a time, provide one utensil, serve finger foods, use aprons to protect her clothing and dignity, serve thick juices and nectars and monitor her swallowing.

Be aware of "chipmonking." This is when a person puts food in her mouth, chews and chews, but can't remember how to swallow, so the food is stuffed in her cheeks.

Chipmonking is a huge choking risk and the mark of the later stages of dementia. When you see this happening, request a speech therapy order from her physician. The speech therapist will feed your loved one a meal and make changes in her diet preparation. For example, she may need her food chopped, chopped finely or pureed. Her liquids may need to be thickened to help her tongue and throat "grab" the liquid to safely swallow.

Be alert to changes in eating styles – fork and knife to fork to spoon to finger foods to mechanical soft to puree is the anticipated routine. Be certain to taste the food before serving and be alert to her changes in taste perception – try sweet BBQ sauce, ketchup, sugar, sweetener, honey, syrup, molasses, applesauce, jelly or jams, etc., to help her taste her foods.

Responding to Resistance: When nothing else is working that day, look for causes and triggers for her resistance. Pay close attention to her cues, and try responding to her emotions. Expect to have to redirect her and try, try again. If all else fails, try singing and praying with her during care. Use a soft and gentle approach and give her lots of praise and reassurance, every step of the way. If she is getting physical, wear a heavy jacket or use towels to protect her and you, especially if she tends to bite, scratch, grab or hit. If she kicks when you walk in front of her, then don't walk in front of her.

Remember the person you love is functioning with an impaired brain and that is the reason for the behavior. You can adapt your behavior. The person with dementia cannot.

Challenging, Combative or Aggressive Behaviors include: arguing, accusing, annoying, biting, cursing, fighting, frustration, threatening, grabbing, hitting, hostility, physical attacks, kicking, pinching, resentfulness, resisting, slapping, spitting, suspicions, and verbal attacks.

Triggers and Causes of ADL Challenges

Physical – She is too hot, too cold, has untreated pain, an infection, her medication (taste, choking, effects are fading), she might be hungry, thirsty, she needs to toilet, her clothes may be uncomfortable, etc.

Emotional – She has depression, loneliness, misses friends and family, and is more confused about her new "home." She may have an inability to recognize home, or to communicate effectively. She may react to "strangers" asking "Do you know who I am?"

Environmental – Her surroundings may be too stimulating, too hot, too cold, too noisy, too quiet, or there may be too much stimuli, the room may be too bright, too dark, or it just doesn't appear familiar, etc.

Task – She may have been asked to do something too complex, too confusing, she can't remember all the steps, she's embarrassed by her inability to remember, chore, social setting, etc.

Communication – She can't understand all the words, or she can't speak well enough to get you to understand, She may not be able to hear you, she can't see you, or the caregivers may have unfamiliar accents, etc.

If your loved one is exhibiting challenging behaviors, remember to check for delirium first. Run through the following list to see if there are any other clues to the changes.

- **First – Identify the behavior**
  - Did something or someone trigger the behavior?
  - What happened immediately before the behavior occurred?

- What were you doing and how did you react?
- Try to remember and answer: What, Where, When, Why and How?

- **Second – Explore potential solutions**
  - What are your loved one's needs? Are they being met?
  - Can adapting the environment help reduce the difficult behavior?
  - How can you change your reaction or approach to the behavior?
  - Are you responding in a calm and supportive way?
- **Third – Try different responses**
  - Did your new response help?
  - Do you need to explore other solutions or causes? If so, what can you do differently?

Suspicious Thoughts Are Part of Dementia

- Don't take offense.
- Don't argue or try to convince.
- Offer simple answers.
- Switch her attention to another activity.
- Duplicate items if lost. Duplicate favorite clothing.
- Stay calm. Breath. Step back and out of sight for a moment.

- Listen to her frustration. Listen to her emotion.

- Apologize, apologize and then apologize some more. A simple "I'm sorry" can do wonders.

Repetitive Actions Can and Do Occur

*Respond to the emotion, not the behavior. Accept the behavior and work with it.

*Turn her actions or behaviors into an activity.

*Stay calm and be patient. Engage her in an activity.

*Answer the person, even if you have to repeat it several times. And then you may have to repeat it several more. It is the dementia causing this behavior, not your loved one trying to annoy you.

Other Tips

*What time of day is behavior occurring? Is it afternoon, morning, evening, nighttime, during ADLs?

*What was the weather? Thunderstorms affect people with dementia. Cold weather can trigger arthritic pain of old broken bones. Hot weather can quickly dehydrate. Remember to stay ahead of the pain.

*Who was around? Is the person reacting to a certain staff member, or is there an unprofessional staff member?

*When is medication due? Is a behavioral medication in use, but its effects are wearing out before the next dosage is due?

*When was last bowel movement? Is the person in pain from impaction or constipation?

*What color is urine? Brown, discolored or strong smelling urine is a clue to check for a Urinary Tract Infection (UTI).

*Is the behavior new or different? Is the behavior a progression of dementia or delirium? Remember dementia is a slow progression: delirium is rapid and requires immediate medical attention.

*Has behavior changed dramatically in the past few hours or days? Check for infection ASAP!

*Is the behavior risky? If the behavior is annoying and not risky or endangering to anyone, then so what? (Cursing for example, may be offensive, but it is not physically harmful.)

*Is the person just having a bad day? (We all have bad days).

*Is the behavior a danger to the person or others? If yes, seek medical attention.

*Did you forget your social skills and trigger an insult response?

*Is the person visually or hearing impaired in addition to dementia? Did you raise your voice to accommodate the hearing challenge and appear to be threatening to the person?

Knowing the answers to these questions help you the caregiver, the physician and medical staff and ultimately, the person with dementia.

⌁

Five Points To Remember:

1. Our behavior can trigger her challenging behavior. And we are the only persons who can change our behavior because she is just responding to her disease.

2. Look for the cause of the behavior, address or change the cause. Remember to treat the behavior and find the cause. Remember, she will not appear sick until the end of the disease.

3. Medications, weather, pain, stroke activity, etc., can all trigger behavior changes.

4. Some dementias will be challenging because of the area of the brain that's affected.

5. Persons with dementia may be suspicious, that's not unusual.

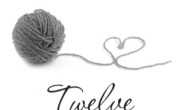

Twelve

STAGES OF DEMENTIA

The destruction of the brain that takes place with many dementias, including Alzheimer's, typically follows a systematic, progressive and recognizable path through the brain. Today researchers have a much better understanding of the function and purpose of the brain than they did just a decade or two ago. And while medical science has not completed its breakdown of brain function, we have determined specific areas of the brain appear to be responsible for specific behaviors.

We also know when these same areas of the brain are damaged a person exhibits these behaviors. This greater understanding of the brain and its functions allows us to be better able to place the behaviors exhibited by a person with dementia into a timeline that tracks the disease's progression.

Being able to track the progression of dementia is critical for all families. First, awareness and understanding of what the disease is doing and which part of the brain is affected allows caretakers to understand the behaviors they are witnessing are not deliberate but are the direct result of damage in the brain.

Again, this is a key factor for all caregivers to grasp, because for much of the disease, your loved one doesn't look ill. Second, the dementia-caused behaviors offer clues to where an individual is in the disease process. This gives a family the opportunity to prepare emotionally for the next decline as well as financially for the costs of providing continuing care.

Many geriatric professionals have used the Global Deterioration Scale (GDS), published in 1982 by Dr. Barry Reisberg and his colleagues, as a framework to track and measure the progression of the disease in an individual. At a time when very little was known about the progression of the dementia, the GDS was the most reliable tool aging professionals had when working with patients and their families. Its seven disease levels provided a framework of the functional decline of the body's systems and helped professionals better understand the progression of the disease and track how the dementia was progressing.

One problem with the GDS is distinguishing between the different levels can be challenging for families and caretakers who do not have a medical background. Over and over I have seen families have difficulties understanding why something called the "late confusional stage" happened before "early dementia." Or why "dementia" wasn't used as a diagnosis until the person had lost significant brain tissue, skills and function.

So in 2009, after more than a decade of hands-on experience with persons in all stages of dementia, I began to develop the Dementia Behavioral Assessment Tool (DBAT) as a way to make tracking the decline of a person diagnosed with dementia easier for both families and professionals.

The DBAT focuses on behavioral changes that typically occur in a person with dementia and then assigns an approximate timeline for each stage. These behaviors are hallmark features of decline in the brain's cellular structure and function, These behaviors also indicate that the disease process has now moved into a certain area of the brain, otherwise these features would not be present.

For example, urinary incontinence is most often seen in Stage Five of the disease process. Accusations of theft are most often seen in Stage Five of the disease. No longer appearing to recognize the presence of others is a feature of Stage Six. Incontinence of the bowel is also a Stage Six behavior and so on. The DBAT also incorporates recommendations and changes made in April 2011 by the National Institute on Aging about the way dementia will be diagnosed and treated.

As we go through the different stages, you'll see I have assigned an estimated range of time to each stage of dementia as well as an estimation of the person's mental capabilities. For example, a person determined to be in early Stage Five has the mental equivalent of an 8 to 12-year-old child while a person in late Stage Five has the equivalent of a 4 to 8-year-old-child. As you look at these timeframes, remember the following important points:

- Not all persons will move through the stages of dementia at the same rate of time. Just as each of us are human and follow a unique progression from infancy to adulthood, those with dementia will each experience slightly different disease progression.

- The progression from one stage to the next is subtle and takes place over time. People don't go to sleep in Stage Five and wake up the next day in Stage Six. Instead, most people experience a back and forth of behaviors until the brain becomes too damaged to recover any earlier abilities and the next stage is now the daily stage.

- Not all persons diagnosed with dementia will live to its final stage and die from the disease. Estimates indicate the majority of people with dementia will die the way most of us do – from a heart attack, stroke or massive infection such as pneumonia.

Predicting how long a patient will stay in a specific stage is difficult and often varies based on the individual's own health. A dementia person in good health who suffers from no additional medical complications, such as hypertension, renal failure or cancer, will be expected to move sequentially through all the stages. This is often referred to as "The Slippery Slope." The differences among individuals will be in the time spent in each stage, not in stage itself. This person will experience all stages of the disease should she live to the end of dementia.

In addition, the type of dementia someone has will determine whether the person moves through all stages progressively (e.g., Alzheimer's and most dementias) or skips stages because of the very unique differences of some forms of dementia. Someone with vascular dementia, for example, may suffer a stroke so severe that she skips one or more stages instead of continually declining on a daily basis. This type of progression is referred to as a "sidestepping the slope."

This name is applied because the person has a significant decline in her abilities and her cognition, and then she stabilizes before the next major health event causes another major decline in abilities. Persons who have Parkinson's disease-related dementia, Lewy Body dementia or Frontotemporal dementia also may experience a decline in the later stages that is more rapid and dramatic than Alzheimer's.

In the rest of this chapter, you will find certain behaviors listed in the DBAT that are unique to each stage. These are the behaviors I have most often seen in persons with dementia, regardless of the type of dementia, in skilled and assisted living dementia facilities.

As you read them, just remember these two important points:

1. Not all patients will display all of the characteristics for each specific stage; rather in some people you may see only a cluster of behaviors.

2. The stages often overlap as the brain struggles with the disease process.

The Start of Dementia

It was believed for decades a person who began to show dementia symptoms, most typically Alzheimer's Disease, in her mid-60s was suffering the effects of a disease that had started only a few years earlier. Experts now generally agree the dementia process may actually begin in a person's 40s. (If you are forty and worried about this, please go see a neurologist.)

The symptoms simply go unnoticed because of the complexity of the brain's structures, its ability to reroute around damaged tissue, and create new pathways for information. This "plasticity" feature of the brain allows the brain to continue attempting to adapt to the damage and the person to continue to function normally for years. Remember how your organs are formed to function above 100 percent? Perhaps the brain does this as well.

One way to imagine the beginning of dementia is like this: I start with 100 billion brain cells. If I damage one hundred thousand or even one million, I'm still okay. If I damage 10 million or even 100 million, I'm probably still okay. But if I damage one hundred thousand every day for months or years, then the consequence over time is that I have a severely impaired brain structure. I will be unable to function without assistance.

In this long, slow beginning of dementia, a person's spouse, family and friends usually do not recognize that anything is wrong. If they do, they may attribute the person's changes to stress, lack of sleep, family challenges, job responsibilities or "normal" aging. Many people in the early stages of Alzheimer's and other dementias often go undiagnosed or are incorrectly diagnosed.

In earlier stages of the disease, dementia can be subtle, the overall changes missed as the medical focus may be on one outstanding feature. Other times features the family thinks may be dementia, may actually be caused by dozens of other disorders – from infections and illnesses to vitamin or hormones imbalances to depression. These symptoms of these disorders can have the same signs and symptoms as dementia. The bottom line is that the earliest signs of dementia are hard to pinpoint, even for professionals.

Certain dementias are now recognized as having an even greater possibility of being misdiagnosed. Lewy Body may be misdiagnosed as depression, addiction or Alzheimer's. Frontotemporal Dementia (FTD) may be treated as alcoholism or another addiction before the dementia is recognized as the true culprit. For persons with FTD and Lewy Body, it is estimated at least three incorrect diagnoses will be made before the disease is correctly identified and treatment begins. For these families, getting a diagnosis in these types of dementia can be an ordeal requiring great faith and persistence.

Stage One: Normal Aging and Cognitive Impairment

As we get older, we know who we are and where we are. We are alert and understand time and concepts. We understand relationships between people, objects and environments. We are able to provide care for ourselves. Our thought processes are logical, and our cognition is intact and operating normally.

Most of us will live and die knowing who we are and experiencing only the normal forgetfulness that all human beings exhibit. Unfortunately, normal aging isn't as appealing to the public as dementia, so there are not many books around about the topic.

Type of Changes

We identify where a person is on the Dementia Behavioral Assessment Tool by looking for changes in cognitive, affective and physical abilities.

- Cognitive changes are shifts in perception and awareness.
- Affective changes are shifts in emotions and feelings, and shifts in how emotions are shown on the face.
- Physical changes are the observable alterations seen in a person's physical condition.

Stage Two: Mild Cognitive Impairment (thought to last 5 to 20 years)

Stage Two is the actual beginning of cognition changes. Known as "benign forgetfulness" on earlier scales, this stage is now recognized and diagnosed as mild cognitive impairment (MCI). MCI may also occasionally be referred to as mild neuro-cognitive impairment. The signs at this point are subtle and may not even be noticeable to most family members.

Cognitive changes include subtle and gradual memory loss, especially of recent events and new information. Other cognitive changes you may see include:

- Uncertainty and hesitancy in initiating behaviors and actions.
- Lessened ability to perform simple tasks.
- Increased loss of reason, logic and judgment.
- Difficulty focusing attention or a decreased attention span.

A person in Stage Two generally does very well in social situations and in normal, nonspecific social conversations.

An example of a nonspecific social conversation would be one that begins with a standard greeting such as, "Hello, how are you?" The reason this conversation is not affected is because we have been trained from the time we learned to speak to automatically respond to that particular question and dozens more like it.

And since Alzheimer's typically destroys the brain's memories in a reverse order, this long-term memory of social skill knowledge is retained and used until the end stages of the disease when speech is finally lost. Only when you ask a very specific question, such as age, year, date or events from the past week or day, (i.e. what was eaten for dinner, who called on the telephone), will you begin to see indications of cognitive impairment.

By the end of Stage Two, cognitive changes may cause a person may begin to perform less effectively at work. She might forget to complete tasks that were once part of her daily routine, she may be unable to add or subtract correctly, and she may have difficulty organizing times and dates. Poor performance may put her in jeopardy of retaining her job.

Affective changes often are seen as a noticeable personality change and may include:

- Decreased interest in one's environment and daily affairs – a type of social withdrawal.

- Indifference to the normal courtesies of social life, including aloof or haughty behavior, and a lessening of facial emotion.

- Gradual loss of initiative, spontaneity and sense of humor.

- Growing absent-mindedness and inability to concentrate.

- Carelessness with appearance, especially in a normally fastidious person.

- Signs of emotional instability, especially depression and anger. (Person becomes depressed because he is aware he is forgetful; exhibits frustration and anger because he cannot remember or do things in the way to which he is accustomed).

Physical changes are, for the most part, nonexistent. The vast majority of individuals show no weight loss or other physical signs of illness until the later stages of dementia. If someone does exhibit outward signs, there may be only some slight weakness or slower movements, or a small amount of muscle twitching. Unfortunately, because a person simply does not look sick, family members often mistakenly think that individual is simply acting out or making life difficult on purpose.

For reasons we don't yet understand, most people try to hide the disease in the earlier stages. People in this stage appear to be aware that they are having memory difficulties that go beyond normal aging. However, if questioned by family members or a physician, they will frequently exhibit an appropriate interest and concern about the symptoms beginning to present themselves, and then quickly dismiss any concerns.

They usually are very good at concealing and compensating for deficiencies. For example, your loved one may use humor to answer questions that are confusing. This humorous response can mislead friends and family into thinking the patient is actually quite with it, so they'll laugh off the forgetfulness. But if you continue to question the person to give you a correct answer, you may frustrate your loved one and get an angry outburst.

This early stage is especially challenging for family members as they try to determine if the occasional slightly unusual behavior they catch glimpses of is normal aging or the beginning of Alzheimer's disease. In many cases, only a qualified neurologist who specializes in dementia, a geriatrician or a geriatric psychiatrist is able to make this diagnosis.

Also keep in mind that today's medical guidelines dictate that a physician must make a person aware of his or her Mild Cognitive Impairment diagnosis and the risk for continued cognitive decline. A physician may choose to begin prescription medication at this point.

Finally, remember a diagnosis of MCI is not a necessarily a death sentence or a dementia sentence. As medications improve and people work harder to stay cognitively enriched, the decline may continue to be slow and subtle. For many persons, the disease will not advance beyond this point, especially if appropriate medications are started immediately. Some studies indicate that the earlier use of dementia medication increases the likelihood of death from old age rather than dementia.

Stage Three: Beginning Dementia (may last 1 to 4 or more years)

Dementia signs, symptoms, and behaviors begin to magnify by Stage Three of the disease. Many family members become fully aware their loved one's memory loss and decline in intellectual functioning is too pronounced to be normal aging. For the individual, the cognitive changes taking place during the middle stages of dementia mean the loss of ability is slowly becoming the norm.

The key word here is "regular." The problems or challenges seen sporadically in Stage Two are now beginning to appear more frequently, though the person may have days of absolutely normal behavior. You also may see an individual fluctuate from one stage and to another throughout the day, as many of the brain's pathways and personality traits remain intact and undamaged.

Although many family members are relieved to know that a relative has an actual disease, difficulties can arise when one or more family members refuse to accept the diagnosis. Denial is not uncommon as dementia comes on quite slowly. When this gradual presentation is added to the Western culture belief that older people become befuddled as they age, some family members simply choose to avoid the topic or to ignore the evidence.

Another area of family conflict that often crops up at this point has to do with medical and financial decisions about how to care for a loved one. This is where knowing what stages and behaviors are to be expected and how long each stage will last becomes especially helpful.

While family members may disagree about how to proceed, she is likely growing increasingly unaware of her problems. She does not always recognize that she has made errors in conversations or lost her train of thought. If she does recognize any of her cognitive issues, she may begin to deny deficits and take greater measures to hide or disguise them. She may increase her use of humor to deflect lapses.

Unfortunately, as in Stage Two, the use of humor is seen by many family members and concerned friends as a sign of cognitive ability. Confused families think that because their mom can make fun of herself or use humor to avoid answering a question, then she must be fine. Those individuals who do begin to accept the fact that they are sick may accept reassurance from caregivers but also will show more signs of depression and withdrawal.

In this stage, changes in perception and awareness grow more obvious as memory loss and forgetfulness begin to impact everyday life, including social, family and job relationships. Forgetfulness will noticeably be more than normal, and you'll see increased confusion when your loved one is in both unfamiliar and familiar situations.

Additional cognitive changes you see may include:
- Difficulties finding correct words and names: She may misuse a word, substitute one word for another, or be challenged to remember the names of new acquaintances.
- Lessening ability to follow and participate in conversations: She may have difficulty understanding a story or a joke, or expressing her own stories and thoughts. She could lose her train of thought in the middle of the sentence. Conversation topics may be inappropriate in relative to

others taking place. Responses to what is being said to her may be wrong. For example, she may answer "yes" or "no" to questions instead of participating in a full discussion.

- Disorientation to time or place: She may get lost on the way to or from work, the grocery store or other familiar places, or she arrives at a scheduled destination at the wrong time or even the wrong day. She may forget an invitation to an event and then accuse family and friends of not including her.

- Needing to constantly check a calendar or make lists: If you are a list maker, this is not an indicator that you need help. Some people naturally make lists, and some professions teach list making as a tool. What we are talking about is making lists where lists wouldn't normally be made, such as lists with the names of children or grandchildren.

- Slowness or an inability to complete a regular task: Everyday routine chores, such as cleaning the house, paying bills or mowing the lawn, will take longer. She may pay the same bills several times over or not pay bills for three months. She may spend all day making dinner, but forget to serve several courses. If still driving, she may have more mishaps with the car, such as denting a fender or getting into minor accidents. These accidents may be blamed on the carelessness of others, or she may not remember how she got dents in the car.

- Poor judgment in making decisions: She may begin to start sending money to questionable charities or she might be giving money away to friends, relatives or even total strangers. She may change her manner of dress. This might be seen in unmatched clothing, no jacket when it is cold or too many layers when it is hot.

- Increased instances of misplaced or lost valuable and everyday belongings: She may be unable to find common items (i.e., keys, shoes, jewelry, broom) even though they may be their proper place.

- Lessened ability to retain information: She may have difficulty remembering telephone numbers, keeping track of money or checkbook balances, and retaining information when reading a book or passage. She may be unable to follow simple directions when driving or walking. She may forget what she was just told to do at work. She may forget where she parked the car.

- Noticeably more affective changes related to emotions and mood: Many children remark that a parent is "not the same" – that their parent may appear withdrawn and disinte-rested and has lost her spark of life. They report their parent has lost initiative to start new things and has lost her spontaneity.

Additional affective shifts may include:

- A more flaccid facial appearance that sometimes seems detached, uninterested and vacant.

- Increased mild to moderate anxiety and more self-consciousness of her behavior. Your loved one probably is aware at times of her symptoms and inability to interact appropriately in social settings. This leads to avoidance of people outside the home and a withdrawal from activities in an attempt to skirt contact with people.

- Wide mood swings along with increased agitation and belligerence that are not usual behaviors.

- Unexpected increases or decreases in a person's sexual desires or behaviors.

Physical changes are not quite so obvious at this point as the disease is still essentially outwardly invisible. You may begin to see signs of poor coordination or balance, and some individuals begin sleeping more than usual or have a change in their normal appetite.

Stage Four: Moderate Dementia (may last 1 to 4 or more years)

If any family members were still in denial about the dementia diagnosis, they should have no doubt as their loved one moves into and through Stage Four. In this stage, symptoms grow more pronounced as the brain's disintegration continues. Estimates are that by the end of this stage, a person has lost several ounces of brain tissue. This is the stage during which you'll need to prepare to provide a higher level of supervision for your loved one as she begins to move into Stage Five.

Cognitive changes, especially regarding recent memories, are greatly affected at this time. For example, you loved one may:

- Not remember visiting family or friends immediately after they leave.
- Forget appointments and socially significant events as well as those she actually attended.
- Forget to initiate or complete normal routines, including health and hygiene measures.
- Report losing more items and expresses mild concerns that those items were stolen.
- Increase repetitive statements or questions because she does not remember what she recently said. This repetition will be noticeable by even those who are not close to her.
- Have more problems recognizing close friends, neighbors and family members, including spouses and children.

- Have problems with writing and reading, although she may hold a book or newspaper and appear to be reading. If she is able to read words and sentences, chances are that she will not be able to fully comprehend the meaning.
- Not be able to recognize numbers or perform math calculations.

Individuals in Stage Four also exhibit increasing challenges understanding or expressing language. They have greater difficulties organizing thoughts, thinking logically and finding the right words. They may easily lose a train of thought, hesitate with verbal responses and make up stories to fill in blanks. This making up of stories is known as "confabulation."

When the brain can't find the pieces of a story it needs in one memory file, it will search for something from another file to fill the hole. Thus, the dementia person may appear to be making up stories when the brain is just trying to function with the files not yet destroyed by the disease. For family members, confabulation may appear to be deliberate lying, especially as a person doesn't look ill and can have long periods of time (hours or days) with no apparent cognitive decline.

Cognitive changes also may include hallucinations and inappropriate social behaviors. Or she may begin to use curse words despite an inability to carry on a regular conversation.

As discussed earlier, curse words are stored on the right side of the temporal lobe (along with singing). Since formal language on the left side of the temporal lobe is destroyed first, she is left with singing and cussing.

Bathing

A fear of bathing is common in dementia and may begin during this stage for some people. This could happen for a variety of reasons. One may be rooted in a sense of survival. Getting wet means getting cold, getting cold means getting sick, and getting sick means dying. Another reason may involve a general confu-sion regarding the challenges of bathing, as it is one of the most complex of the activities of daily living that we perform.

Other reasons may be a sense of modesty, a feeling of shame for needing help, an inability to understand a caretaker's accent, a feeling of being insulted or just an overall feeling of poor health that day. People with dementia are allowed to have "bad" days too.

Affective changes also increase at this time, as damage in the brain means the dementia person is less able to main control over her emotions. Emotions run the gamut at this stage and can fluctuate wildly, and a person may appear to have the emotional responses of a hormonal teenager. For example:

- One minute she may become suspicious, irritable or angry; the next minute she may be fidgety, teary or silly.
- When she laughs, she may laugh too loud or too long for the situation.
- When she is upset, she may get very agitated and upset.

At this point in the disease process, your loved one may begin to slowly have an increased dependence on significant others. She may experience adult-child role reversal and become socially isolated and withdrawn. Behaviors consistent with depression may be common and should be addressed by a qualified physician specializing in dementia behavior.

Physical c hanges, including poor muscle coordination resulting from apraxia, become more apparent in this stage. Although apraxia can affect healthy older adults who don't maintain an exercise regime, the type seen in persons with dementia is different. A normally aging adult needs to continue to be mobile to maintain balance and function.

A person with dementia loses balance and function because of damage to her brain. As her gait becomes less steady, she is at a higher risk for falls. You may witness more repetitive movements, muscle twitches and jerks as well as more perceptual motor problems like difficulty understanding how to move her body with or around an object. In other words, she begins bumping into tables, chairs, etc., with her body.

Additional physical changes beyond the increasing lack of coordinated movements include things such as:

- Increased appetite for junk food and the food of others while not appearing to notice her own plate of food. Some dementia people report being very hungry even though they just ate, because the person may not remember that she just ate.

- Damaged internal nocturnal clock that causes confusion between night and day. Finding a loved one restless or aimlessly wandering at night is not unusual. Neither is witnessing a slow and gradual increase in sleeping, especially during the day.

- Lessened ability to attach meaning to sensory perceptions. A winter storm's cold or summer's heat may have little meaning. The sound of a warning siren may go unheeded.

- Increasing loss of facial emotion expression. Your loved one may frown more, appear annoyed or angry, or have little facial movement.

Final Stages

The last three stages of dementia are extremely difficult to watch as your loved one loses more abilities and moves closer to death.

If you haven't already looked for help in caring for your dementia person, now is the time. By Stage Five, she likely will require the type of nursing care and 24-hour monitoring provided by a qualified dementia-skilled nursing home or dementia-certified assisted living community. For most persons, Stage Five is when a dementia diagnosis is finally made. At present, the estimated average time before death is five years at this stage.

Stage Five: Moderately Severe Dementia (last 1 to 3 years)

In the beginning of Stage Five, a person's abilities are the equivalent of someone between ages 8 and 12. By the end of the stage, those abilities are closer to a person who is 4 to 8 years old. The individual also will have lost approximately one-half pound to one pound of brain tissue by the end of this stage. In other words, because of the disease, the brain will weigh closer to two pounds instead of the three pounds of a health brain.

In this stage, a person can no longer survive without some assistance but will still appear and act normal for short periods of time. In fact, an outsider or family member with little contact would have difficulty believing this person has serious cognitive difficulties caused by severe brain damage. This person still looks physically healthy.

An individual will wear clothing and supportive appliances, such as dentures, hearing aids, eyeglasses, jewelry, scarves and hats, correctly. Women will carry a purse, and men will carry a wallet. Most individuals are still capable of conducting non-specific social conversations.

This stage is particularly frustrating to caretakers for a couple of reasons. First, are the challenges facing family members. Some caregivers will grasp that mom has significant problems. Those siblings or family members who only rarely talk to or interact with the person who has dementia may be less receptive to reality.

For example, a daughter living out of state may believe the once-a-week social conversation she has with her mom via a telephone call is a realistic reflection of her mother's abilities. The out-of-town daughter believes her mother when mom says she takes her medicine, visits with others, attends church, etc.

Meanwhile, the daughter providing daily care sees an entirely different level of abilities. She knows mom is missing medications, gets lost in the neighborhood, has to be reminded and driven to the doctor. These two different views can cause great conflict between the siblings as to the parent's true condition.

Second, a person at this stage may begin to be resistant to care giving. Most typically, this is because she does not believe she needs assistance from others. Her ability to perform the activities of daily living remains relatively intact, but supervision is beginning to be needed for eating, toileting, and bathing, grooming and dressing. Her ability to use humor to answer the out-of-town daughter's questions is incorrectly interpreted as cognition and not confusion.

Cognitive changes in Stage Five are exhibited in a number of ways as memory deficits steadily increase. For the most part, this person still has a sense of awareness but seems lost in time. In other words, she will have knowledge of past, present and future events, but lack a full appreciation for what those events mean.

For example, she may know her children are coming to visit next week but confuse the current week with that future one. She also will likely have disorientation about time (year, date, day, week, season) or place. It is important to remember that this person can score very well on a Mini Mental Status Exam, but not on a cognition test.

An individual in Stage Five also retains knowledge of many major facts regarding herself or others, but may be unable to recall major aspects of her current life. So although she'll likely remember where she was born and the names of her spouse and children, she may not know the names of her grandchildren or the address or telephone number of the home she has lived in for many years.

She may, towards the middle or end of this stage, speak about her parents or other long-deceased relatives in the present tense. For example, she might describe herself as a young wife and talk about how her mother frequently visits to teach her how to make a piecrust.

Sundowning Syndrome

You may also begin to see an increase in a behavior called "Sundowning." Sun-downing, or active wandering is when an individual exhibits a strong desire to leave her current home or community, generally in the early or late afternoon for a specific purpose, such as a need to feed her children or visit her sick mother. Another feature of Sundowning is that the person may believe she actually lives somewhere else and insist that she is just visiting her current residence. She may talk about going "home" to place where she raised her family or the house where she grew up as a child. Although this behavior is most strongly associated with Stage Five, some report seeing it during Stage Four as well.

What Is It?

Sundowning Syndrome remains somewhat of a mystery in gerontology and is an endless source of frustration to caregivers. Some persons with dementia, regardless of the type of dementia, never experience Sundowning. For others, this is a daily struggle for caregivers. In many instances, the person with dementia will attempt to leave the current environment regardless of weather, time, safety issues or reality.

In earlier stages of the disease process, (Stages Three, Four and Five) a person with dementia is able to verbalize a reason to leave, such as picking up children, returning "home," going to work, etc. This is referred to as "purposeful wandering." In other words, the person can state the reason she needs to leave.

Later in the disease, she may still attempt to leave, but due to the advancement of the disease process, can no longer state a reason. Once a person can no longer articulate to others where she is going, she is exhibiting a phenomenon called "purposeless wandering." This form of the behavior is normally associated with the later part of Stage Five and Stage Six.

There are several theories that exist for Sundowning including restless leg syndrome, agitation, fatigue, or noticing there is a change in staff around three or four p.m. In my opinion, Sundowning is more realistically tied to an innate human behavior that is hardwired into our evolution.

Since humans began, we performed a number of tasks throughout the daylight hours, but as the sun began to move into the lower sky, we stopped the day activity, moved to another area and begin to prepare for the evening and nighttime.

Think about it like this: cavemen stopped hunting and returned to the cave, farmers stopped farming and returned to the cabin, and in your own lifetime you have lived within the same timeframe.

As a child, you were aware a parent came home in the afternoon/evening, a meal was prepared and then bedtime occurred. School started and you became actively involved in these events. You left school to return home for the evening. As an adult, you probably continued this pattern; you left work and returned home. Or if you stayed at home, you stopped your daytime activities and begin to prepare the evening meal, etc.

Sundowning is simply the human brain continuing this evolutionary behavior. The difficulty is when the person with dementia has difficulty realizing and recognizing that he or she is already home and another person is performing those previous tasks. The challenge for caregivers then is how to address Sundowning in a manner that's the least stressful for everyone involved, the caregiver and the person with dementia.

Tips for Sundowning

1. For the majority of persons with dementia in Stages Three, Four, Five and Six, design activities that allow your loved one to use up energy during the day. But remember these

physical activities, such as dancing, walking, exercise, etc., need to take place in the morning (10 a.m.) and in the afternoon (around 2 p.m.). Starting the afternoon activity after 2 p.m. appears to help increase Sundowning, rather than burning up energy that would be used in Sundowning.

2. Other persons react better to earlier physical activities (10 a.m. and 1 p.m.) and then respond positively to an afternoon "nap." Remember the nap needs to take place in an area other than the bedroom, as waking up in the bedroom can further confuse your loved one into thinking it is morning time again.

3. But because humans are unique, other persons react negatively to too much activity. Caregivers are tasked with finding which schedule works best for their loved ones.

4. During the day, keep the home or community as well lighted as possible. High wattage bulbs, all lights on, blinds pulled, etc. to allow maximum daylight helps your loved one stay better acclimated to day activities.

5. Should Sundowning begin, look for activities to engage your loved one. This might mean a walk, music, a favorite movie, helping with a task, or rubbing lotion on the hands, paying special attention to the palm area. (This is often a soothing activity).

6. If your loved one becomes physically aggressive, back away from her and try to reduce noise and movement in the environment. If she is agitated by your presence, try stepping out of her sight for several minutes. (Make certain your loved one is safe however). You might even try to change your shirt or hairstyle before your re-approach, at times this change in appearance will result in a change in behavior.

7. In the event your loved one is able to leave the home, keep a recent photo and medication list handy and do not hesitate to contact the authorities. Remember a dementia alert bracelet can be ordered from your local pharmacy and can be worn on the wrist or ankle.

Additional cognitive changes in people in Stage Five may also include:

• An increasingly limited ability to participate in social conversations is noticeable in this stage. This person will be able to function fine for several minutes to half an hour or more, but then begin to repeat her conversation and statements. This is because immediate memory (about five minutes) is impaired while speech and language skills are still functional. Many in this stage typically will enjoy reminiscing conversations about times when she was younger. This is because those files are still intact, and the brain can pull memory from those files in a way that allows her to be involved in conversations.

- Difficulty counting backwards. This skill shifts from an inability to count back from 100 by 7s to an inability to count back from 40 by 4s to an inability to count back from 20 by 2s, even for highly educated individuals.

- Use of tactics to disguise memory deficits. Social skills are still relatively good, so a person may use humor to sidestep a question requiring more detailed knowledge or higher cognitive ability.

- This same individual also may become argumentative, upset or combative if pressed to answer questions beyond her capabilities. She may look to her caregiver to supply the answers too.

- Impaired language abilities. Estimates are that a person in this stage understands three out of four words in conversation.

- Increasingly delusional, suspicious and anxiety behaviors related to short-term memory loss. She may now begin to forcibly and angrily accuse family members or caregivers of theft when she doesn't remember where an item has been placed. (Note: In some cases, your loved one may be correct, so check to make certain an accused person is not doing these things. Abuse of the elderly, especially demented elderly, certainly exists). She may accuse a caregiver of attempting to harm her because of confusion about the activity being performed. Bathing, for example, can be interpreted as an assault or attack.

- Perception of reality is based on misperceptions. She may, for example, continue to believe she still has responsibilities that are work or family related.

Affective changes also increase in Stage Five and may behaviors include:

- Tearfulness, depression and catastrophic outbursts can occur daily or weekly.

- This person retains her own agenda and insight into situations. Her beliefs about her surroundings are very real to her, regardless of how nonsensical the caregiver may perceive the situation. Her reality is your reality.

- Increased sensitivity to environmental stimuli that prompts negative or challenging behavior. Too much background noise; too much movement, or too many people, cars or city lights can be upsetting to someone with dementia. Shouting can be misinterpreted as anger and cause someone to be physically or verbally combative or protective of her space.

- Hunting and gathering activities. In a community, residents will wander in and out of each other's rooms while they look for things they have "lost." A person may collect jewelry, shiny items, stuffed animals or any other number of items and not want to give them back. To safely retrieve an item and avoid combative outbursts, try trading for something different or distract her with cookies or another treat rather than simply taking the object away.

- Increasing depression. A person at this stage is still aware she is losing her abilities and may admit to being afraid because she can no longer remember her family. She also may express that she believes she is a burden to others and that she wishes to die.

Physical changes are now more evident than ever before as motor skills and balance continue to decline. The risk of falls increases during this stage. You may also see the following:

- Despite increasing coordination challenges, your loved one may still be able to use the toilet most of the time although she may need reminders to use the commode and assistance getting there, dealing with clothing and sitting down or getting up. However, incontinent episodes will begin to occur as her body begins to fail to send or recognize signals from the brain when it is time to use the bathroom. Eventually incontinence becomes a weekly event and then a daily event before the ability to toilet one's self is gone.

- Your loved one will start to perform repetitive activities that are physically soothing. Examples include folding cloth items such as napkins, tissues and towels. She may perform this activity for hours or at different times throughout the day.

Stage Six: Severe Dementia (lasts 1 to 3 years)

As a person moves through Stage Six, her brain will be destroyed to the point where it weighs between 1-1/2 to 2 pounds. This person will respond to her environment with the ability of a 2- to 4-year-old child. Interactions with her will reveal a serious loss of abilities.

Cognitive changes are fully evident, as a person is generally unaware of her surroundings in terms of time of year, season, month or day of the week. In the beginning of this stage, the individual will retain some knowledge of her life, but the information recall will be sketchy at best. With less than five minutes of short-term memory, she is largely unaware of recent events and experiences. Instead, she'll be better able to remember events that took place much earlier in time and will discuss them as if they are occurring in present time. These discussions will be greatly impacted by a severe loss of language abilities during this stage.

Additional cognitive losses in your loved one at this stage reveal the following:

- The individual will continue to be able to distinguish familiar persons in the environment but be unable to recall names properly. She may forget the name of her spouse and adult children as well as the caregiver upon whom she is entirely dependent upon for survival. She may continue to know her own name.

- She will have difficulty counting forward from 1 to 10.

- Speech and language deficits are more pronounced. The individual will not be able to think abstractly or comprehend that she is having deficits, and will have great difficulty initiating or engaging in conversation. She will, however, usually retain social skills although the use of them is rudimentary. This means a person at this stage will be unable to converse after standard social pleasantries are exchanged. Any conversation she does make will tend to be social clichés that she uses without really understanding the meaning of them.

- If the person is multilingual, she will revert to the language she first learned when growing up.

- She will no longer recognize or be able to use common objects, as agnosia is complete at this point. Because she does not recognize items such as eyeglasses, dentures, hearing aids, splints, braces and Band-Aids or their purposes, she will remove them and either throw the objects away or hide them away in drawers, closets, shoes or other places.

Affective changes are more pronounced in this stage, and you can expect more frequent personality and emotional changes. It is not uncommon that your loved one will exhibit the following:

- Delusional and obsessive behaviors. For example, spouses will be accused of being an imposter or she'll repeatedly perform cleaning activities, such as wiping a tabletop. This behavior will cease towards the end of this stage.

- Increased anxiety, agitation and violent behavior (even if the person was non-violent in the past). These behaviors are a result of cognitive impairment that causes an individual to be unable to carry a thought long enough to determine a purposeful course of action.

- An insistence on completing activities her way.

- A complete lack of sense of personal responsibility, including no concern about her whereabouts.

- Increased hunting and gathering behavior.

- Fear of being alone. This person will frequently search for social contact. If she has moved to a facility, she may confuse another resident with an old friend and spend most of the day with him or her, even though she is unable to make conversation.

- An unkempt and haggard appearance with a face that looks flat and devoid of expression. She will appear disheveled within minutes of being "fixed up."
- A refusal to change her clothing and a tendency to frequently layer clothing.

Physical changes continue to speed up in Stage Six. At this time, the deterioration of the brain causes the dementia person to:

- Be at greater risk for falling. The ability to coordinate muscular movement and coordination is further impaired and, at the end of this stage, posture, gait and balance are seriously impacted.
- Become totally incontinent and unaware of the need to empty her bladder or bowels.
- Lose peripheral vision and depth perception. Visual interpretation problems and their associated behaviors are more pronounced in this stage. This is the time when a person is easily startled by people, bumps into more objects, taps the floor with her foot to test it and seemingly pinches the air in front of her.
- Have disturbed sleep patterns. A person may sleep during the day and stay awake through the night, or may require

16 or more hours of sleep and then stay awake for 18 or more hours. Some individuals will stay awake for two or more days at a time before requiring sleep. Another person may fall asleep during meals or while doing activities.

- Either restlessly pace, refuse to walk at all or even remember how to walk. If she tells you she can't walk, even though she could this morning, she is not trying to make your life difficult. She can't walk at this time, her brain can't figure out how to maintain balance, place one foot in front of the other, stand up, etc.

- Require assistance with all activities of daily living. When a caregiver tries to help, the dementia person may become aggressive or combative.

Stage Seven: Very Severe Dementia (may last 1 to 3 years)

In this last stage of dementia, the effects of amnesia, aphasia, agnosia, and apraxia have almost run their full course in a person. By the end of the disease process, the brain that once weighed three pounds will shrivel to only one pound, and the individual moves from the ability of a two-year-old to that of a newborn. Cognition, affect and physical changes are so significant that the your loved one will no longer resemble the person you knew before the dementia began its painful toll on her personality and her body.

At this point, an individual's cognitive activity is now very low. In Stage Seven, speech and language deficits make it impossible for the person to initiate conversation or interactions with others, and her attention span will be extremely short. Although your loved one cannot carry on a conversation or comprehend spoken language, she may show awareness of simple gestures, pantomimes, facial expressions, familiar musical tunes, environmental sounds and the emotional tone of your voice.

She may utter a few non-meaningful words or non-words. Responses to painful stimuli may be expressed with some sort of vocalization or may not evoke any response.

You also can expect an individual in Stage Seven to:

- Not know her parents' names or recognize any of her family members, including a long-time spouse.
- Be unable to recognize or use common objects.
- Be unaware of danger.
- Attempt to remove her clothing regardless of the temperature and fidget when sitting or laying down.
- Seek immediate sensory gratification if something looks, tastes or feels good.

Affective changes are dramatic. At this point in the disease, a person's affect is almost nonexistent, and her eyes will have a vacant look without focus. Your loved one may experience visual or auditory hallucinations even though she is unaware of her surroundings. She could become even more resistive to caregiving or may be totally placid in an almost semi-comatose state.

Physical changes are dramatic as well and appear much faster than in the previous stages. In addition to looking extremely ill, your loved one will:

- Experience significant weight loss. Remember that as the brain deteriorates, your loved one will forget she is hungry or thirsty and will eventually forget how to chew or swallow food.
- Drool more as the swallow reflex diminishes.
- Exhibit (early in the stage) hyper-oral activity where she may place anything, including trash and feces, in her mouth.
- Suffer significant posture changes, including losing the ability to walk, hold up her head or maintain balance when sitting. She will not be able to get out of bed at the end of the disease. She may even be able to have great flexation in her body; that is she can cross her legs and pull her knees up to her chest, her hands will appear to curl up, turn at the wrist and her arms will bend at the elbow and tighten. It does not

mean she can be moved easily however. With flexation, she must be treated with great caution and gentleness.

- Lose her ability to see the environment around her. Everything will appear flat.
- Sleep 20 hours or more per day.
- May have seizures and because of her bed bound state, she will be at great risk for skin infections or skin breakdown.

The last ability your loved one will typically lose before she dies is the ability to smile. This can occur a few months or a few weeks before the process of active dying begins. At the end of Stage Seven, death takes place, as the brain can no longer tell the body how to sustain life.

Five Points To Remember

1. **Dementia follows rather predictable stages of decline and deterioration. Some persons steadily decline, others appear to have stable periods followed by sudden changes in abilities.**

2. **The seven stages of the Dementia Behavioral Assessment Tool provide a way to track the decline of a person diagnosed with dementia.**

3. People move through the stages are different rates, so determining an exact timeline is impossible.

4. The stages are not independent of each other and the progression from one to another generally overlaps.

5. Not all persons diagnosed with dementia live to its final stage. Most people who have the disease will die from other health reasons earlier in the disease process.

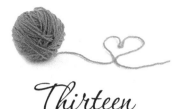

Thirteen

ACTIVITIES AND DEMENTIA

You have probably realized by now that because your mom is losing her abilities in a reverse order, caring for her changes dramatically. Your day may seem as though you are caring for a 150-pound adolescent, then a 130-pound toddler and finally a 115-pound infant. The scale that tracks this decline in dementia is known as the Alzheimer Retro Genesis Scale -- literally the "back to the beginning" scale.

As your loved one loses her ability to be active doing the previous hobbies, games or social skills she loved, you will need to keep these changes in mind, so you can adjust how to provide meaningful activities for her.

Just make certain that although she may appear to act and think like a child, she is not a child, but an adult with an acute brain disease. No one is allowed to talk or treat her as though she is an infant. Especially in a skilled facility or a memory community.

Your loved one deserves to be addressed by her name and not a pet name. She should not be referred to as honey, baby, grannie, girlfriend, etc. She should be treated with the respect due an elderly person or an adult.

Bake Some Cookies

So as you think about having activities for her, use your skills and her history. Let's take a person who loved to cook. Let's say for example that your mom was a cookie baker. She has always made cookies.

You remember coming home from school and she would have fresh chocolate chip cookies coming out of the oven, just as you got off the bus. She has spent a good portion of her lifetime making cookies for sick friends and neighbors, parties and holidays, for picnics and church luncheons.

But dementia has taken away her ability to make cookies. At first you might have noticed her measurements were off, too much salt for example, or the cookies were slightly burned. And then you realize she has stopped making cookies altogether. When you ask why she may tell you she is no longer interested, or she doesn't like cookies anymore. She may even use humor and tell you cookies make you fat, so she stopped baking.

In reality, she is no longer doing this favorite activity because she can't remember all the steps required to bake cookies. Measurements, ingredients, turning the oven on, the right temperature, the right time in the oven, etc. are all part of a complicated set of steps.

Just like bathing or toileting, her files and memories on baking are also becoming damaged. The process is overwhelming to her now, or she's afraid she won't be able to bake the cookies right.

Now remember dementia has not stopped and she is going backwards in time and ability. In the beginning of Stage Five, she is the equivalent of a 12-year-old, then an eight-year-old and by the end of this stage, a four-year-old. So how would you help children in these ages make cookies?

For the 12-year-old you might have the ingredients, measuring cups, spoons, etc., out and ready. You would monitor the oven and the baking times.

For the eight-year-old, you might help with measuring and give even more assistance. For the four-year-old, you will be providing a greater level of guidance. Perhaps at this stage she is only stirring the cookie dough.

For a Stage Six person, more help from you will be needed. And a Stage Seven person might just enjoy being around you and enjoying the smell of the cookies baking, while you make the cookies and remember past holidays spent cooking.

The activity, whether it is baking cookies or playing cards or painting, planting flowers, or doing exercise, is based on the stage your loved one is in and how much assistance she will need. The same way you would make allowances for a child, or provide extra guidance, you will do again for your loved one.

Dominoes, for example, may become a game of matching fives or a game of matching numbers. It might slowly turn into a game of clacking the dominoes around and the sensation of them under her hands. The games may be longer than usual or shorter than before. The point is the enjoyment of your loved one playing a favorite game. It is the tactile feel of the dominoes, the social time spent with you, the familiarity of the game that matters.

Memory Boxes

Memory boxes are great ways to have little activity sessions for the busy caregiver without a great deal of fuss or muss. They are called memory boxes because each one has a theme and items inside related to the theme. Once each type of box is set up, you simply give any one of the boxes to your loved one and allow her to open and explore.

Common themes might be "sea shore," "animals," "wedding day," "army," "family photos," "spices," etc. The box then contains items related to the theme that are safe for your loved one to touch, smell, wear or taste.

A sea shore box might contain coconut lotion, a bottle of sand, photos of the sea or a family vacation, a lei necklace, sea shells, a coconut, whatever you can think of that would remind her of the ocean. Getting out the box and discovering the contents allows you to have an activity that might trigger old memories, or fun stories.

Your wedding box might have rice, wedding photos, a flower, wedding veil, or any number of items your mom might recognize. It lets you talk with her about her marriage, her first date, when she fell in love, or how she met your dad.

An easy way to make this at home is to use old shoeboxes. Label each one with the theme and make certain to use them. Who knows, you might discover a memory you didn't know before!

Exercise

Daily exercise is important for everyone, but just like baking cookies, it changes over time. Early on, you might find walking is an enjoyable activity. But later, balance or weather or recovery from an illness might mean trying to create an exercise routine indoors. This can be simply walking up and down the hallway or around the house several times or doing chair exercises.

As dementia continues, mobility might be a real risk factor for your loved one, so you might try chair exercises. These include everything from lifting your feet while seated as though you are walking to doing stretching exercises or using small, one or two pound hand weights.

Try to make these exercises vary by adding a story to each one. Stretching exercises might involve a tale of going to the country and picking fruits and vegetables. To pick an apple or a peach or an orange for example, means having mom reach and stretch her arm, grab the apple and twist her hand to pluck the apple from the stem and put the apple in the basket. Each time she picks an apple, she also counts aloud to give her lungs some exercise as well.

Chair exercises are fun ways to keep in shape and maintain her range of motion. For you the caregiver, the exercise also helps you relieve stress and stay in shape. Many of these types of exercise are available on DVDs. In earlier stages, your loved one can follow along without assistance, but in later stages, she will need you to help her along. In the final stage however, her exercise will involve only gentle range of motion exercises, as she will be extremely frail and fragile. These will vary from person to person, so be certain to check with her physician for guidance.

If you begin to feel overwhelmed or think you don't have activities in your home for your mom, think again. The following is a list of activities that can be done in 30 seconds or less and anyone can do them. Ready?

Tell her you love her, greet her by name, make eye contact and smile, hug her, shake her hand, give her a compliment, notice a bird or squirrel outside the window, give a hand massage, try on a new shade of lipstick, play a quick game of catch with a balloon or a soft ball, share some hand lotion, smell cinnamon, blow bubbles, ask her an open-ended question, slip her a piece of candy or chocolate, share a photo on your phone, ask for advice on a recipe, look at a flower arrangement and talk about the colors, tell a joke or funny story, ask about a childhood pet, ask about her first kiss, sing a song together, say a pray together, or make her laugh by doing a quick dance step.

There are lots of other activities around the house you can enjoy with your loved one. Keep a basket of black and white socks for her to sort and put together. Or keep another basket of washcloths for her to fold.

We aren't certain why, but sorting and folding are enjoyable activities, as is wiping off a kitchen or dining table. The motion and movement appears to be soothing and helps her feel needed and productive. People have a need to feel useful, needed and wanted. Watering the ivy plant, giving the dog a treat or folding washcloths are all helpful in this respect.

Other activities you have around your house include things like: read a short story or poem, plant seeds, listen to favorite music, pop popcorn, have a cup of tea, finish famous quotes, play Old Maid, color a picture of the flag, cut up fruit, smell spices, make toast and jelly, name the presidents, wind yarn, sort cards by colors or numbers or suits, sign favorite hymns, watch old TV shows, make Jell-O or pudding, look at baby pictures, try on funny hats, put together a simple puzzle, play trivia games, clip out coupons, polish shoes, snap beans or clean beans, sing together, give a manicure, take a walk, decorate cookies, have a spelling bee, play hangman, feed the birds, plan a party, or you might even roll pennies. The point is that activities are all around us!

Most families and caregivers are not aware of the variety of activities that are available in our homes. You can also try planting a basil, sage, rosemary, thyme, etc., herb garden as a sensory activity. Just pluck a few leaves and smell. Also, a few sprigs of rosemary in a vase next to the bed appear to be calming for some persons as a sleep aid.

Make the activity fun for you and your loved one. And be creative. I know of one community that routinely has a really fun game. The residents roll dice to score the number they have selected, say a "five." Every time a five is rolled, each person gets a Hershey kiss! You get the idea?

Persons in Stage Six of dementia are more difficult to engage in activities. To do so frequently requires more one on one care, as they are easily distracted. In this stage, the person is withdrawing into her own little world and is not really interested in what we are doing. However, a favorite activity can continue to engage her when all else fails.

Mary's Story

Mary was the wife of a pastor. She had been the music director at each of their parishes and was a gifted and talented pianist. But in Stage Six of Alzheimer's, she could no longer play her beloved piano or remember her hymns. When a familiar hymn was played, she would cock her head slightly, as if she was trying to recall the words, but she had stopped speaking several months before. Instead she would hum along, the words seemingly just out of her touch.

She was beginning to lose weight. Sitting at the dining table was a chore for her. Anxious and agitated, she would grab food in her hand and quickly move away. Once she learned

I kept candy in my pocket, she would suddenly appear and stand quietly waiting for me to notice her.

It was not hard to miss her at times. Like many people with advanced dementia, Mary would move only inches from me and stand. Once the candy was unwrapped and in her hands, she would give a small quick smile and she was gone again.

Her agitation and withdrawal made it difficult for the staff to engage her in activities of any kind. If there was no music, she wasn't interested.

One day, we noticed her sitting quietly by the piano. Just staring off into space, she had a peaceful look on her face. It was as though she was waiting for the church service to start. Now I am not a pianist, but Mary was so still in that moment, I had to try.

A caregiver had placed a CD player on top of the piano. Small and dark, it was barely noticeable behind a pot of flowers. I opened the player and couldn't believe my luck! The CD was church hymns, accompanied only by a piano.

Turning the CD player on, I sat at the piano and moved my hands over the keys in time to the music. Mary never sang a word, but we had discovered her activity. Every afternoon, a different caregiver would sit at the piano, turn on the CD player and move her hands across the keys. Mary never sang a word, but just sat quietly nodding along, her foot keeping time, her hands folded perfectly across her lap.

The activities in Stage Seven of dementia are different. Because of the advanced decline of the person, tactile and sensory activities are most often used. These include CDs of outdoor sounds, birds singing, waterfalls, oceans, rain, winds in the trees, favorite music, lotions, scents, soft materials, etc.

Activity Pillow

As persons in later stages of dementia become more tactile and less mobile, an activity pillow can be a blessing. While you can purchase pillows online, it is not too complicated to create your own.

This design calls for a pillow measuring about 13 x 18 inches. That size will fit neatly across a person's lap and is pretty standard for an accent pillow, so it should be easy to find at the store. Look for one that is brightly colored and has a soft texture. Remember tactile means touch and you want something very soft for your loved one.

If you are not a person who sews, you'll need to find a friend or tailor to assist you. On one corner of the pillow, you will need to sew a cord long enough to tie to the handle of a wheelchair or side chair. This is so when your mom gets tired of the pillow and tosses it off her lap, it won't fall on the floor and be a fall hazard.

Make certain all of the items you sew on are very tightly sewed on because persons with dementia do not lose their strength. And since she will fiddle and fiddle with the pillow, it will take quite a beating.

So you have a soft, nicely textured pillow and a long cord sewn to one corner. Next pick out a few baby squeeze toys at the store. They will be something like a small dog or rabbit or fish on a string. These are small stuffed animals that allow you to pull on them and then the toy will make a noise or vibrate. You can find these in the baby section of any store.

You are going to sew these stuffed toys onto the pillow. Remember to use extra stitching, as this item will be used.

To assemble your pillow, place the pillow on your lap. So if you are looking down at it, image the pillow is like a clock. You would sew one toy at 12 o'clock, one toy at 3 o'clock and one toy at 9 o'clock. Placement of these toys and the three dimensional quality of the toys means your loved one will have a greater chance of seeing them.

Don't forget to wash your pillow and watch for worn stitching. Most families report they made at least two and sometimes three of these for their loved one.

Baby Dolls

Some of you might have noticed by now that baby dolls are usually present in communities. Some even have entire nurseries, complete with blankets, carriages or bassinets, bottles and clothes. It is recognized that persons with late stage dementia -- usually Stages Five, Six or Seven -- are very much drawn to babies. They like children and they treat dolls as though they are living babies.

This need to nurture is very real, and for this reason, it is recognized that some people with dementia benefit from having a baby doll. Most states have a regulation in the nursing guidelines that only a person with a dementia diagnosis is allowed to have a doll. The guidelines further state the attending staff must treat the doll as real whenever they are engaged with the person.

The dolls can be a very real asset and activity for your loved one. Just be aware that these dolls get a lot of loving and have to be replaced rather often as they get quite worn. Also remember if your loved one needs a baby doll, you will need to collect it from her before meals, as she may be too attached or worried about the baby to eat herself.

Five Tips To Remember

1. A person's abilities to perform the many dozens of steps in an activity decline with the disease.

2. The selected activity must be altered to fit the abilities of the person's stage of dementia.

3. Stage Five persons can generally follow along during activities and Stage Six persons require one-on-one assistance.

4. Persons with dementia may enjoy having a baby doll as an activity.

5. Activities should be based on the person's prior interests and hobbies.

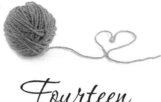

Fourteen

CARING FOR THE CAREGIVER

When a loved one is diagnosed with dementia, one adult child or parent or spouse generally becomes the primary caregiver. You may find yourself shouldering most of the burden, especially if other siblings live nearby, yet don't, can't or won't help out.

You are a caregiver if you do any of these tasks: cooking, dispensing medications, transporting and arranging for medical appointments, housework, personal care (sleeping, ambulation, toileting, hygiene, grooming, dressing, eating) or doing the banking, shopping, cleaning, laundry, bill paying needs, and any legal needs.

If you are the caregiver, chances are pretty good you are dealing with a high level of stress, anxiety and/or depression. This possibility increases if you are over the age of 60. If you have been a caregiver for more than three years, you can also add an increased risk for high blood pressure, increased colds and flu, chronic pain and even fibromyalgia. All of these are the result of the stress of caring for a person with one of the dementias.

How we react to changes in life determines to a great extent how our bodies will adapt. Do you see the diagnosis of dementia as positive, because now you have a confirmation of the behaviors and cognitive changes you've witnessed?

Or is the illness itself too much of a negative? Any change in our lives is a stressor, and for caregivers, the stressors can seem to increase every day, with little or no apparent break. For many caregivers, the stress goes on for years.

Making the challenge of caregiving more difficult is that so many of you are alone or isolated, without support or respite. How do you deal with what stress is doing to your emotional and physical self?

Take a Deep Breath

Let's start with a simple breathing technique that takes only a few moments to complete and will reset your autonomic nervous system. The ANS is part of your internal systems and affects your heart rate, digestion, respiration, and your fight, flight or freeze responses, even the increase of blood flow throughout your body. Resetting the ANS happens instantly when you do this technique.

Now if you have difficulty meditating, feel silly trying to still your mind, or as a caregiver, just don't have the time, this exercise is perfect for you.

Breathe in slowly through your nose to the count of six. Simply count one, two, three, four, five and six and then slowly exhale through your mouth to the count of four -- one, two, three, four. Repeat this same breath count, in through the nose while counting to six and exhaling through the mouth while counting to four -- three more times.

That's it! In less than one minute -- really for many caregivers all the time you might feel like you have -- and like magic, your autonomic system resets and your tension is gone. The ease of this exercise means you can use it as many times a day as you need to and in the process, calm your heart, blood pressure, settle your stomach and maybe get through the rest of the day.

With practice, you can increase the amount of time you do the breathing exercise. Some people are able to work up to ten minutes of breathing to reduce their stress; other caregivers try the technique in its shortened form (four breaths) several times a day.

Remember, you are under a lot of stress. Do something nice for yourself. A bubble bath, a cup of tea, order a pizza, have someone come over so you can take a nap, call a friend. You are doing the toughest job there is, remember to breathe!

Finding Help

If you find you are alone as a caregiver, look for other options. If you have other family members, call a meeting. Schedule a time to meet with all of your siblings or involved family members to discuss your loved one's needs.

Make an agenda for the meeting. It will make everything easier. Write down the details of how you feel in a matter-of-fact way. Family members may not be aware of how you are feeling. Remember they may be feeling angry or hurt about being left out or they may be feeling guilty because they are not helping.

Be specific about what you need. Do you need a respite break, to vent, help with appointments, meal preparation or shopping? Divide up the tasks, even among family members who live faraway. Several family members pitching in a little money can pay for a caregiver for a few hours or visit every few months to give others a break.

Don't be afraid to ask for help, but be realistic. Old family wounds and slights are probably not going to be made better by this, but then again, maybe someone will step forward to help.

Look for outside agencies as a resource. Start with the federal government's Area Agency on Aging. This agency was formed during the Older Americans Act in the 1960s. The case managers and other employees are skilled professionals who can direct you to care, or depending upon your area, may be able to provide some respite care. They will also be aware of any church respite groups and any other programs available where you live. And they cover all areas of our country.

Find a support group! This is critical to your frame of mind. The Area Agency on Aging also offers teleconference support groups for caregivers who are homebound. These telephone calls allow you to dial into a conference, which usually lasts about an hour, listen to professionals discuss some topic on caregiving, talk to other caregivers and never leave your home. It can be a lifesaver to just talk with another person who understands what you are going through.

There are also caregiving groups that meet online if you have computer access. You can use You Tube to find caregiving videos to find the answers to specific concerns or questions about care you might have.

Another important thing to remember is dementias are diseases that eventually require medical care and assistance. You have not failed your loved one if you need to seek outside placement. Most people don't have large families anymore and many families are scattered around the country. It doesn't make you a bad person when you need to find other care options. Just remember the cancer example. If this was cancer, you would make certain your loved one received the needed medical care. Dementia also requires medical care.

Tips for Dealing with the Family

1. Use e-mail reports to keep everyone on the same page. This leads to less confusion and everyone gets the same information.

2. Use conference calls to connect all interested parties. Most physicians are glad to contact out of town or out of state family members and explain details of care to them.

3. Make a list of the main points you need to make for this call and stick to the list.

4. Call when there is an issue; don't just expect everyone to know what's going on. Remember, everyone grieves differently; no one way is right or wrong.

5. Prep your relatives for upcoming issues. Let them know a doctor's appointment is scheduled for next week and then try to follow up with the results.

The Keys to Successful Aging

As you find yourself drawn into full-time care, remember you have to stop and take care of yourself. Many times when I see a person with dementia, the caregiver is in worse condition. Frequently, the caregiver is exhausted, mentally, and physically.

Tips for Dealing with Yourself

- Look at old photos – place photos in an album, use new computer books to add stories to photos or use a digital frame to upload your favorite pictures and enjoy the show.

- Inhale calming scents such as orange and lavender, or enjoy a piece of cinnamon toast and a cup of tea. Baking muffins, bread or cookies makes us smile.

- Open your shades to increase light your home, replace low wattage bulbs with higher watts and keep the lights on during the day. It really helps!

- Walk outside. Just take a walk around the block or to the end of the street. Light exercise increases the heart rate by 40 percent and makes your brain and body feel better.

- Clear away the clutter. Straighten up piles of papers. The illusion of order eases the mind and reduces anxiety.

- Think fast. Spend 30 seconds thinking positive thoughts. It'll make you feel better.

- Google information that interesting to you. Use the Internet to look up information. It lights up the brain, and it is free.

- Cue up YouTube and watch funny videos, or your favorite old (funny) movies. Remember, your brain likes eating, sex, and laughing. Laughing is free! These activities increase dopamine and make the brain happy!

- Put on a happy face and stand up straight -- good posture and a smile lead to positive social interactions.

- Zone out, daydream, and reminisce. It is good for you. Give yourself a timeout, kick up your feet, close your eyes and think about something fun.

- Chat up a friendly neighbor. It increases the chances that you'll be happy too!

- Chop up your veggies. It is a favorite unwinding exercise and you can create a wonderful soup or other yummy dinner. And chopping vegetables allows you to zone out and relax.

- Do a good deed. Volunteer with a group or help one person. It'll make you feel good to help others! In spite of all my good intentions to help you breathe, contact the

AAA for assistance. Caregiving can still kill you! Chances are you go to the doctor pretty frequently, but I'm betting it is rarely for yourself!

Below is the Caregiver Burden Scale. This is a measurement scale designed to alert family caregivers to the amount of stress and physical danger they are in as care providers. Take a few minutes to honestly answer the questions and count up your score. If you are over 40, please contact your doctor! Repeat the test every couple of months as stress levels change as the disease progresses.

Caregiver Burden Scale

Rank these statements on how true they are for you as a caregiver, using a scale of 0 to 4 with 0 = Never and 4 = Nearly Always.

☐ I don't have enough time for myself.

☐ I am over-taxed by my responsibilities.

☐ I have lost control over my life.

☐ I am uncertain about what to do for my loved one.

☐ I should do more to help my loved one.

☐ I could do a better job caring for my loved one.

☐ I feel burdened by caring for my loved one.

____ **Total Score**

☐ My loved one needs help all of the time.

☐ My loved one depends on me to help her complete her daily tasks.

☐ I fear what may happen to my loved one in the future.

☐ I fear that there will not be enough money to care for my loved one.

☐ I fear I will not be able to continue to care for my loved one.

☐ I wish someone else would take over my caregiving responsibilities.

☐ I feel a sense of strain when I'm with my relative.

____ **Total Score**

☐ I sometimes feel anger toward my loved one.

☐ I am sometimes embarrassed by my loved one.

☐ I feel uncomfortable about having friends over.

☐ Caring for my loved one has a negative impact on my relationships with other family and friends.

☐ Caregiving has affected my health.

☐ Being a caregiver impacts my privacy.

_____ **Total Score**

_____ **Total points from all scores.**

Interpretation: No or Minimal Burden: 0 to 20

Mild or Moderate Burden: 21 to 40

Moderate to Severe Burden: 41 to 60

Severe Burden: 61 to 88*

Adapted from The Family Practice Handbook

Five Points To Remember

1. **Caregiving causes your Autonomic Nervous System (ANS) system to function poorly.**

2. **Breathing exercises or other meditative activities can be very helpful.**

3. **Call a family meeting to ask for help.**

4. Check with your **Area Agency on Aging** for assistance or guidance or to get started with professionals dedicated to giving care to the persons in their community.

5. Take care of yourself. If something happens to you, who else will be there to provide care? What you do is so important.

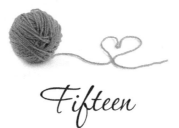

Fifteen

The Final Year...The Final Moment

We have a hard time with death in our culture. You may even find it difficult to say the words "death" or "died" or "dying." And you wouldn't be alone. As demographics have changed and more and more people live in urban areas, fewer of us are exposed to or witness death.

Death has become an unknown thing, a frightening apparition. Aging and the process of death are foreign to us, things to be avoided at all costs.

Perhaps we don't say these words aloud because of their power. The finality of death brings an end to a relationship. The loss of a loved one, cherished relative, or friend is so hard to bear. Your pain is exposed and naked for all to see. Or perhaps, it is because of a society that places more value on youth and very little on age. After all, 50 is the new 40, right?

On a farm or ranch, children learn about death early. Whether it is the loss of a newborn kid goat, calf, or lamb; a cheeping baby chick that disappears in the night; or the sudden dispatching of a predator, country kids see death often. They grow up exposed to life endings that are brought about by the process of living, illness, or old age. After all, death is a part of life, and ironically enough, the natural end to all creatures.

But times have changed us. Death, even the expected death of a loved one, even a death you may have prayed for due to the ravages of dementia or another disease, causes us to pause. It takes our breath away, makes us physically ache.

Most of us no longer live in an agricultural setting. And in a society bursting with knowledge about life, relatively little study or research is focused on death.

Men are socialized to act differently when confronted by the death of a loved one than women are. And we are socialized to treat men differently. For example, we expect women to cry and men to be strong. Whether the death is a man's parent or his child, outsiders will comfort the daughter/mother more than the son/father.

It is not uncommon following the death of a child for example, for persons to inquire as to how the mother is doing, but not ask about the father. Likewise, the death of a parent or spouse or even a father-in-law or mother-in-law is rarely seen as impacting the son/son-in-law. We just don't seem to "get" that the deceased may have been just as loved by the son-in-law as if he/she was a parent.

Such societal mores make the man's grief process even more complicated. Just remember whenever someone dies, everyone in the family is affected, everyone is grieving.

The Modern Death

It is estimated in the course of our current lives, each of us will witness death only once, maybe twice. Those deaths will most likely be of a loved one. You may be sitting with a beloved grandparent, parent, spouse or even your own child when death arrives.

The months, weeks and hours leading up to the moments of a final breath can be confusing, frightening and may shake your faith deeply. Our own lack of information regarding the final moments of life can greatly conflict and compound the mystery and fear that often accompany death.

Among people who work with the dying, a demand for the dignity of the person's final months, weeks or moments is often forefront in care planning. The recognition we as professionals need to respect a person's wishes, whether it is for "full code" care, meaning that all medical measures will be utilized, or if it is for comfort and palliative care, or for a Do Not Resuscitate order (DNR), does not waiver.

Even if the care a person or their family chooses may be contrary to what we know medically about the probable outcome, or if those wishes collide with what we would want for in our own lives, respecting the wishes of each person, is vitally important.

For some persons, the dignity of their death may be simply wanting to be allowed to be included in discussions about their pending death. To be able to admit death is coming is a powerful thing for the person dying. Talking about the pending death is difficult; indeed it feels almost impossible when you're involved in the conversation.

Just remember the elephant in the room doesn't get smaller or go away. You may even be surprised to find having that conversation is the most positive and powerful thing you can do in an otherwise hopeless situation.

For others, it may be the way we address them. Some persons may wish for solitude and others may seek the comfort of friends and family.

We estimate about 80 percent of persons die in a medical setting. Following a cardiac or vascular event (heart attack or stroke), a fall or accident, etc., persons are admitted to a hospital for treatment. So death may occur in the hospital. Or death may occur following treatment and/or placement in a skilled facility (nursing home) or a dementia community or hospice facility.

In spite of popular opinion and the most common hospital setting of death, physicians and nurses are rarely in the presence of death. Only ER responders, physicians and nurses routinely see the passing of life. In the rest of the hospital setting however, it is not the job of the physician or nurse to sit with dying persons.

Because of this, there is a clear gap in our medical literature and knowledge regarding the final moments of a person's life. Such examples of the physiology of a death from old age or a long and protracted terminal illness are difficult to locate even in medical textbooks. Because medical training is focused on the procedures to preserve life, rather than the physiology of the cessation of life, the research and literature just doesn't exist.

Physicians are trained to combat death and may even attempt to do so even when common sense says the battle is over. Examples we see most often are additional procedures ordered even though the patient is hours or moments from death, or invasive procedures ordered with terminal end stage illnesses, such as dementia.

Jack's Story

Jack was a man I had known for several years. The time had come and he was dying from Progressive Aphasic Dementia, one of the types of Frontal Temporal Dementia.

He had been ill with the disease for several years. His wife Helen had provided for his care until their children insisted Jack be moved to a dementia facility for 24-hour care.

The entire family was involved in Jack's life and paid close attention when we discussed the progression of the dementia and the expectations of what would occur at the end of Jack's life – the physiology of his final days and hours.

The children had routinely visited their father in the dementia facility where he lived his final two years and they had cried with their mother at the loss of their father's abilities and mind during that time. His grandchildren, from the adults to the newborns visited Jack frequently, the youngest always sitting on his lap, happily patting his face.

A retired minister, Jack had contracted an infection a few weeks before and was now actively dying. His brain, severely damaged by the dementia, could no longer tell his body how to fight off infection. Nearing death, Jack's breathing had become more sporadic.

His wife and children sat at his side, their chairs touching each other and Jack's bed. They held his hands and told him what he had meant to them as a father and husband. Jack's children did this even though he was unable to respond to them. His eyes were half open and fixated, his mouth was open and his withered body trembled with the effort of every breath. They read his favorite Bible passages, prayed together and one by one, told their father "goodbye."

Jack's breathing had changed to abdominal breathing by this time and apnea was present. The stoppage between breaths was at times more than 85 seconds and he had been in this state for several hours. He would expel a breath and then 15, 30, 45, 60 seconds or more would pass and his ragged body would exert itself one more time and he would draw in another breath.

Suddenly Jack's physician entered the room and shooed his wife away from his bedside. She smiled and bent over Jack and listened intently to his chest with her stethoscope. Without any comforting words to the family, she stepped back from Jack's bed and announced she was ordering a new blood test and medications. The lab tech, she declared, would be in shortly to draw Jack's blood from veins already blue and shrunken from his slowing circulation.

She offered no insightful thoughts to Helen; she appeared to completely disregard the plain facts in front of her. Turning to Helen and the children, she smiled -- new medications, more lab work, more tests! As she turned to leave the room, Helen touched the doctor on the sleeve.

"I don't want any more needles stuck in my husband," she quietly said with great dignity. "He's almost gone and we're okay with that. We're here and that's all anyone can do."

As she had supported his ministry throughout their marriage, Helen supported Jack's dignity one last time. She accepted his time had come and sat back down next to her husband. Shortly after 2 p.m., she kissed him goodbye.

The Dignity of Death

The dignity of death is the decision of a family to decide when enough is enough. Research and stories abound of medical interventions ordered time and again for terminally ill persons, procedures that have no possibility of sustaining or supporting life. Did you know we actually spend more money on the care of a person in the final three months of their lives, than we spent in the previous 10 years?

Dementia is a progressive and terminal disease. Unless another medical complication, such as a stroke, heart attack or cancer, cuts life short, a person diagnosed with dementia will most likely die from complications of dementia. And the dementia disease process can take many years.

Those with Alzheimer's disease can expect to live up to 20 years, depending upon when they were diagnosed. But because most people aren't diagnosed until the disease is already quite advanced, it is currently estimated most people die four or five years after diagnosis.

Some move quickly through each stage of the disease; others stay in one stage for years and suddenly take a steep decline to another stage or death. Others seem determined to hang on as long as possible at the end stages.

And anyone who has watched a loved one suffer through the cruel indignities of Alzheimer's or any other dementia and slip away a little bit at a time understands why it is often referred to as "The Long Goodbye."

But we will all experience the grief that comes with death, whether we were physically there at the last breath, or on the other end of the telephone when we got the call.

Thanatology

The study of death, dying and the culture of death is called thanatology. Translated from the Greek, it literally means "speaking of death." Yet in American culture, we are challenged to avoid death or aging at all costs. As a culture, we have difficulty with the realization that death comes for us all and the aging process is something we can only alter with surgery so many times.

We are so afraid of death that even our obituaries only tell us of someone's "passing" or "journey," not that the person "died." I just checked The Dallas Morning News and was not at all shocked to find out only one person died yesterday. The rest passed peacefully, or went somewhere.

This fear of even talking about death impacts us greatly in our loss. Uncomfortable with thoughts or words of death, we find ourselves frozen in our grief and unprepared for the reality of what happens to us when a loved one dies. How do we act, what is normal, how long do we really grieve?

This change in how we view death is a relatively new phenomenon. When my mother was a child, her paternal grandfather died at home, the way most people did in the 1940s. The United States' population at the time was a rural one. The closest hospital was more than an hour away, funeral homes were seen with distaste and distrust, and death after all, was an accepted part of living.

Mother remembers with great clarity that the dining room in her grandparents' house was rearranged for the service. She knows that her own mother washed her grandfather's body and groomed his hair. He was dressed in his Sunday suit and laid out on the dining table for a visitation service from neighbors, friends and family.

A group of sons and other family members sat with his body through the night, talking and occasionally laughing in low tones as they recanted stories of their father. He was buried the following day in a grave his family dug.

But even this homey scene was a dramatic change from when that grandfather was a young boy. While his family mourned his death and received condolences and recognition from others, death at the turn of the century had a different culture. Persons who died then were commonly cared for at home and a service was most likely held in the home, but the dead person was also mourned for a period of a year in a way persons out side of the family could recognize.

Family members would wear black clothing or a black armband to signify the act of mourning and allow others to recognize his/her loss. A broach worn by women would have the deceased's portrait or picture affixed to it. Other common jewelry included a pin to carry a lock of the deceased hair as a sign to others to recognize a family's loss.

Fast forward to today and check the obituaries in the newspaper. As I wrote earlier, it is more common to find that persons listed there didn't actually die yesterday, but instead went on a journey. Some went to see Jesus, some went home to the Lord, some went to a garden, some went to Heaven, some became choir members, the variance is wide.

I don't say this to mock those beliefs, but to point out our experience with death is so rare and so frightening to us, that even when the result is death, we have great difficulty saying it. We use words like "we lost Bob yesterday," or "Bob's no longer with us," or "Bob passed," as if changing the text will change the loss.

I can tell you that for some parents who have had a child murdered or die; the word "loss" can be a fighting word. I once heard a mother reply with great rage that she hadn't "lost" her child, her child was buried at the cemetery, she knew right were her child was. But she continued with a trembling voice, "I didn't lose my child. My child was murdered!"

Cultural Differences

Other cultures view death differently. Mexicans celebrates a "Day of the Dead." Foods and gifts and parties occur at the cemetery and those loved ones gone are remembered and recognized. In some Native America societies, speaking of a dead person is viewed with great concern. The belief is that to speak the person's name may hinder him or her on the journey to the next world or invite bad luck to the living.

In other cultures, the deceased is not mentioned for a period of three days and the room in which he or she died is also not entered for the same three days. It is believed the person's spirit needs time to leave the space and to enter the room or say the person's name interferes with this process.

Grief and Dementia and Death

If you've heard of the stages of grief as described by Dr. Elisabeth Kubler-Ross, a pioneer in grief research, you know she divides the process into five distinct stages: denial, anger, bargaining, depression and acceptance. Understanding the grieving process as you work through the losses that take place as dementia steals away the person you love will allow you to better deal with your own grief and with the grief of others when your loved one dies.

Unfortunately, family members and friends of persons with dementia tend to experience the five stages repeatedly throughout the disease process – going from denial to anger to bargaining to depression to acceptance – before facing a new loss of abilities and another round of emotions. It is as if they are stuck in an excruciatingly slow revolving door where the stages of grief seem endless.

Just as you come to terms with and accept what you've lost in one stage of the disease – a part of your mom's physical presence, a part of your mom's personality – she moves into a new stage, only to have more of her stolen away.

Understand that the feelings of grief felt throughout the dementia process and how each individual deals with those feeling are unique to each person, so don't be too quick to judge others. Visiting a parent or spouse in the late stages of dementia - someone who looks at you with no recognition in his or her eyes - is painful and difficult for everyone.

Some simply cannot face the slow demise, so they arrange for care at a facility and are never seen again. Others visit only when they feel they can emotionally and mentally handle the visit. Others face the disease process daily and continue to stay deeply involved in the life and care of their loved one.

Some families go through the stages of grief so often they can delude themselves into thinking they are ready for the end. But the reality is this: in spite of the grief of ongoing loss and in spite the pain and hurt caused by dementia, you can still walk back into that room and see your loved one until death actually occurs. Only when someone dies are you able to start your way through the final round of grieving.

The Stages of Grief

What follows is an overview of the stages of grief. Remember that one person may experience all five stages; others may get hung up after only one or two. Some people go through the stages in the order listed, other skip around. No one way is better than another, no one way is right. Just know these are the feelings you, your family and your friends might experi-ence when someone loved has dementia:

1. Denial

How family members react when they first hear a diagnosis of dementia and are told their loved one has a terminal disease or death varies greatly. Most people either consciously or unconsciously refuse to accept the facts, information, and reality of the situation as they are thrust in the "this isn't happening to me" stage.

This defense mechanism is perfectly natural. Some in their shock and disbelief decide the medical professionals must be wrong and begin a journey of taking their loved one for second, third and fourth opinions. Others continue to act as if nothing has happened and go about their daily activities as if all is well. Some choose to isolate themselves.

During this initial grieving phase, many report feelings of being numb and out of touch. They don't seem aware of their surroundings, may not feel connected to their bodies and have difficulty concentrating or making decisions.

If the feelings of denial and loss are too severe, they may not be capable of performing of their normal daily activities, such as cooking meals or driving a car. People often report forgetting to eat or driving to a place and then not remembering the route they took or the red lights they passed.

2. Anger

In the second stage, the "why is this happening to me" stage, individuals experience feelings of anger. Some people may find they are angry at themselves, while others may direct their anger outwards and lash out at those closest to them.

Understanding that your own anger and the anger of others is a normal reaction may help you remain detached and non-judgmental, especially when you are on the receiving end of someone's rage. I once witnessed a daughter come into a memory community and angrily chew out the caregiver because of the way her mother's clothes were hanging in the closet. In reality, the issue was not the direction of the clothing hangers. It was the daughter's grieving process.

Anger can manifest in many ways, including:

- Anger at the dementia that is killing a loved one and transforming her into a virtual stranger.
- Anger at those in the medical field for not being able to stop or cure the disease.
- Anger at themselves either for wishing mom's death would come to end the torture of watching her slip away bit by bit, and/or for not having had more patience in the past with their mom's dementia-induced behaviors.

- Anger at the person who has the disease for putting people through the trauma of watching the disease progress.
- Anger (and fear) that dementia could happen to you as well.
- Anger at the caregivers.
- Anger at the person who is ill or has died.

3. Bargaining

The bargaining stage can be especially difficult because nothing can be done to end this disease for a person or bring her back after death. People in this "I promise to be a better person if…" stage desperately pray and offer exchanges in an attempt to change reality. Sometimes they actually are able to trick themselves into believing their exchange will make a difference.

The best way to deal with someone who is in the bargaining stage of grief is to not offer false hope. The reality is that the course of dementia or death cannot be changed.

4. Depression

When people begin to realize the full extent of their loss, they may move into the depression stage of grief. Common depression signs include difficulty sleeping, poor appetite, lack of energy and crying spells. You may often feel lonely and isolated and say things such as, "I just don't care anymore." You may lose interest in activities, feel guilty or have trouble concentrating. You may feel the other side of depression, known as atypical depression, which includes symptoms of feeling angry or anxious.

Although depression is common after a loved one dies, many family members experience it prior to death. Depending upon when a loved one was diagnosed, you or your family may have been dealing with many medical, financial and behavioral issues for years. This certainly increases to probability of depression.

Realize that everyone has limits and sometimes stepping back and taking a break is the best thing to do. So instead of visiting a loved one for an hour that day, a phone call or quick five-minute stop may relieve some of the pressure.

After the death of a loved one, depression is likely to be intensified and may feel like it will last forever. It is important to remember two things:

Depression after someone's death will not last forever.

Depression after someone's death is an appropriate response to a great loss.

For some people, normal depression after a loved one's death can turn into clinical depression. If you suspect that you or someone you know might have crossed the line into clinical depression and is unable to accomplish daily living activities or has suicidal thoughts, seek grief counseling and an evaluation with a mental health professional or your physician immediately.

5. Acceptance

Eventually, most people get to the point where they can say, "I'm ready for what's next." How long it takes to get to acceptance, especially after a death, varies greatly. For many people, the period of mourning and grieving for loss is actually closer to 10 years than two months.

Even if the death was expected and follows a long illness such as dementia, a person still mourns as if death had come as quickly as a cardiac event or in an accident. As people accept the loss and let go of grief, the anger, numbness and sadness begin to go away.

This does not mean that they are okay with what has happened. Instead, this is an acceptance of the reality of the situation and an acceptance to live with this new norm. Acceptance does not mean that the past or the person is forgotten.

Finally, as you deal with personal feelings and the emotions of others who also care for someone suffering from dementia, remember that help is available through support groups. They provide a caring, encouraging, non-judgmental network that connects you to others who are going through or have completed "The Long Goodbye."

In today's world, we normally receive only three days off from work for the death of a loved one. Well-meaning friends usually allow us a few weeks before our grief makes them uncomfortable. Even close friends typically provide only about six weeks of support. Well-meaning friends may even tell us that the death of our loved one was "for the best, after all she had been sick a long time." That may be so, but it doesn't take away the fact that your loved one has died.

Family Responses

Sitting beside dementia patients in their last few hours, I've found that families react to the pending death of their loved one in a variety of ways – none of which is good or bad. For example:

- Some families sit with a loved one around the clock. They made a decision to be there and share in the final hours, minutes and breaths. Like Jack's family, they are together as they cry, laugh, say their good-byes and hold their loved one's hand in the final moments.

- Some families only want to know when it is over. I once called a woman to tell her that if she or her children wanted to say good-bye to her husband and their father, they needed to come to the nursing home that weekend. She thanked me for calling and said they would not be coming to the facility because they had already said their good-byes. She explained that she and her family believed that Harold had essentially died seven years earlier and all that was in the nursing home was the shell from which his spirit had already left.

- Some families react with anger. One time a granddaughter arrived at the facility after I alerted the family that the patient was close to death. This granddaughter declared she loved her grandmother dearly despite never having called or visited during the time the woman was in the facility. She began yelling at the nurse and staff, finally demanding I tell her grandmother to "stop dying immediately."

- Some families react with indifference. I've had families tell me they can't stop by because they are going out to dinner or the movies.

What's important to remember is that what's right for one family, may not be right for another. Every family is different, and has its own history to deal with as death comes closer. That seemingly sweet elderly lady may have beaten, berated and ignored her children and driven them away over a lifetime.

And everyone grieves differently, whether it is wailing loudly, standing stoically without shedding a tear or getting drunk. No individual should make judgments about whether another's reaction to death or grief is appropriate.

The Actively Dying Process

Regardless of the variety of ways in which families respond to a loved one's impending death, people die in a somewhat orderly manner. Many believe that just as life took 40 weeks to form between conception to birth, the body takes about the same length of time to go through the process of shutting itself down to die.

The fact is that, with the exception of a massive stroke, heart attack or accident, most individuals follow a somewhat predictive path toward their final breath. The human body shows signs and symptoms that allow us to track the process of death and to alert families to prepare for the end. Professionals who work closely with the terminally ill call this process "active dying."

As already mention, few people today experience the process of death firsthand, so what actually takes place in the final days and hours of a person's life can be scary to those who don't know what to expect. I've always felt that being prepared for the inevitable and understanding what is happening to your loved one makes saying that final good-bye just a little bit easier.

As you read the next section, keep in mind that these are guidelines and not all people will experience all signs of pending death. The uniqueness that makes each of us different in life also extends to our deaths.

The Theory of the Cycle of Life

Gerontologists have observed that people often die during the time of year in which they were born. That is, people die in the season or cycle of their life.

The theory states that once a person passes the age of 25, he/she is more likely to die within the season of their birth. Before the age of 25, a person is more likely to die in an accident.

The accidents have to do with youth -- the frontal lobes of the brain aren't quite mature and nothing in the body hurts yet. Think about it like this: I'm 51 and you could not possibly "dare" me to jump off the Lake Belton Bridge. That bridge stretches for a mile over the Leon River in Central Texas. It is long, high above the water and scary. But my nephew Dixon thought (when he was 19) that such a jump was a wonderful way to respond to a dare from a buddy.

You and I are pretty sure such a jump would hurt, so we would laugh off the dare. (Dixon has since confirmed it did hurt!)

So according to the theory, because I have passed my mid-twenties, and because I was born in September, my death should take place in August, September or October. My mother was born in the summer, so she should die in the summer.

Thirty days before the birthday and 60 days following the birthday is the time we call "The Cycle of Life." It seems there really is a time to be born and a time to die.

Signs of the Final Stage of Life - Actively Dying

People who are actively dying exhibit certain symptoms that tell us the functioning of systems is slowing and that the time of death is near. Knowing what these signs are can help us say our final "goodbyes" and prepare us for the inevitable.

The following is a compilation of the signs and symptoms we see as someone enters into the final phase of their life. Not every one experiences the same things or the same order, after all we are each unique individuals. These behaviors are reported when medication is not involved and when oxygen levels are unchanged.

Regardless of where a person is from or what their religion is, these are the signs reported from around the world. They are reported when medication is not involved and when oxygen levels are unchanged.

When you begin to notice these signs, especially if your loved one is losing weight or has a terminal illness such as dementia, contact your physician. The doctor will write the order for hospice to evaluate and decide if your loved one meets criteria to receive hospice services. Think of hospice as an extra layer of comfort and eyes, not as impending death.

Hospice personnel are highly trained in the process of comfort care and should be especially aware of your loved ones' needs. They will focus on palliative care, that is, comfort care. A meeting with the hospice team will determine what medications are needed for your loved one and a plan to provide care and comfort medications will be discussed.

Special equipment such as a hospital bed, a circulating air mattress, wheelchair, or additional caregivers will be ordered as needed. Hospice nurses are available 24 hours a day and will be able to assist you in this final time. Medical care for your loved one will be overseen by the hospice physician and the team will work diligently to answer any questions or concerns you might have.

Tips For Care

Hospice Care: These are businesses whose design is to make certain your loved one is being provided with comfort care during the final stage of life. Hospice does not mean death is imminent. I believe it is better for the person and their family to have hospice in place for several months before the end.

Your doctor will write the order for hospice care and then you will be contacted by local hospice businesses. Pick the team you feel most comfortable with, because hospice services are providing the same type of care. Since this will be a set of professionals working with you at a critical time in your loved one's life, make certain you like the people coming to your home or to the community.

Hospice does not mean your loved one will not receive medical treatment. Should she break her hip or develop a cold and require hospitalization, hospice will technically stop while she is being treated at the hospital. You will start hospice care again once she is released from the hospital.

The hospice nurse or social worker will explain the Do Not Resuscitate order and arrange for the order to be prepared. A DNR is different from a living will or an advanced directive.

The DNR means no extraordinary measures will be taken in the event of a person's death. In other words, if her heart stops, she is allowed to die without receiving CPR. Most families don't realize the results of CPR on old, frail persons. Broken ribs can result because CPR is a very powerful compression of the rib cage. Research also indicates persons with dementia who require CPR and are revived; tend to die within three days of the procedure. When the body is ready to die, we might delay the process, but we cannot stop death.

Wound Care

The body must have circulation moving freely. When you see the letter "Q" and the number "2" written about a patient's bed, it means the person must be repositioned every two hours to avoid skin breakdown and a pressure sore. Decubitus ulcers, bed sores or wounds are dangerous, especially to persons with dementia.

They can quickly become septic, meaning the body is overwhelmed with infection. Sepsis can rapidly cause multiple organ failure and death. Remember skin is our biggest barrier to infection.

Critical areas to watch for are any place where skin and bone touch. These include: the back of head, top of spine, middle of spine, lower spine, sacrum/coccyx/tailbone area, hips, knees, heals, and less frequently, elbows and the pinky side of hands. This means your loved one must be repositioned and moved every two hours, even if she is not responsive to sound or light or other persons.

Gently turn her and use pillows to separate her legs and feet and more pillows to keep her on one side and then the other. Set your alarm for two hours and turn her again. This will help keep her from developing wounds.

Wounds can quickly erupt as a person gets closer to death. A wound care RN (registered nurse) will attend to the wound, as it requires specialized care.

Remember:

1. The new dressing should be dated and initialed by the RN each time it is changed.
2. If the dressing is located on your loved one's bottom, it cannot be covered by a bandage and then a diaper.
3. These wounds occur quickly as the result of a lack of movement and circulation. First the skin turns pink (stage one), then it forms a blister (stage two), the blister opens (stage three) and the wound begins to enlarge rapidly and/or tunnel (stage four) into the body.

The Final Months

- Your loved one may begin sleeping more and you may have difficulty arousing him or her. This is normal and indicates your loved one is beginning the process of Actively Dying. Anticipate that you will want to take advantage of periods of greater alertness to begin your own process of saying "goodbye."

- Your loved one may experience a significant change in status around his or her birthday. Often when families look back, they realize that the final year actually began with a sudden and unexplained change, a loss in weight for example. This may or may not follow an illness or any other diagnosed condition. A physical check-up may not reveal any differences, yet families often report "something" seemed off.

- Your loved one may begin to report having clear and vivid dreams about deceased relatives. This is a difficult time and may be a very tearful time for you as it is a marker that the dying process is ongoing. It is a common feature and reported throughout the world.

- This is a time when your loved one may talk about missing a beloved relative, such as a parent or grandparent. Your loved one may talk about longing to see that person again.

- A diagnosis of "Adult Failure to Thrive" is often made. This is commonly used when no other explanation for changes in physical status can be made. The person should be healthy or be recovering from an illness or fall or surgery, yet the decline in physical and mental abilities seems to continue.

- Your loved one begins to withdraw from activities he or she once found pleasurable and may appear less interested in social activities.

- Your loved one may exhibit a noticeable confusion about time and place, the identity of relatives, friends or other familiar people. If you notice this symptom, assist the person by referring to persons in the room by name. Do not question the person by asking, "Do you know who I am?" Identify yourself if your loved one seems confused about your identity and assure him/her of your presence and your love. The confusion will seem different from the loss and confusion exhibited by a person with dementia.

*Any nurse or caregiver should identify herself when assisting your loved one and should also explain what she is doing step by step.

Nannie's Story

*A*nyone who knows me, knows how important my maternal grandmother was to me. I cherished her sense of humor, her insight, and her intelligence. Every moment I shared with her I found to be a brightly wrapped gift.

As I went through graduate school, I delighted in taking my newfound knowledge of normal aging and making the comparisons to her own aging process. She was marvelous as she listened intently to my description of the theories of aging and offered gentle insights into what was sometimes very dry material.

But a fall and a fractured wrist and a stroke started her down a road I didn't want to travel. I clearly remember the October evening, sitting next to her over a snack of cheese and crackers and pickles and sweet tea, when the reality of her journey became evident even to me.

My beloved Nannie began to tell me how much she missed her mother, how she had been dreaming of her and longed to see her. My great grandmother had died of complications from a stroke when Nannie was only 26. I knew her photograph hanging in the hallway, the dark haired, dark-eyed woman, but I had never heard Nannie talk about her mother.

I felt my heart clutch with each word. I seemed to know what she was going to say before she even said it. The worst part was, I understood what it meant. Nannie was going somewhere and nothing I could do or say was going to stop her.

My grandmother died on a cold December day, only a few days before her birthday. A couple of days before, she had become very alert and she asked us wrap her in a favorite quilt and carry her outside to her garden to sit. Even though she could see the garden from her bed, she needed to breath the crisp air and watch the birds dart through the bare trees one more time. And even now, a decade later, I cry as I write this, so strong is my grief.

The Final Weeks

Frequently, families report that their loved one is no longer making eye contact with them, but instead is looking above them and appears to be seeing or talking to someone else. This is a phenomenon of the process of dying/death seen and reported in every culture. Some people believe this is the reaction to the brain's decreased amount of blood flow and oxygen. Others believe it is because the souls of loved ones are present and ready to guide your loved one to the other side.

Your loved one may report seeing long dead grandparents or parents or other favorite persons calling to them. If your belief is that this is the soul preparing to go with loved ones, then this behavior can provide great solace and peace.

Your loved one may reach out as though he or she is trying to touch someone. He or she may have conversations with people or things not visible to others. Or he or she may report talking to family members who are already dead.

Your loved one may also report that he or she is talking to people who are telling him or her to "Come on."

Your loved one may report strange feelings in his or her limbs. As the person enters more into the final stages of actively dying, he/she may experience a loss of sensation, power of motion or reflexes in the legs and then the arms.

Your loved one may begin to tire easily or talk less and his/ her voice may weaken easily. Avoid tiring your loved one by expecting him or her to actively participate in conversations for long periods of time. Holding his or her hand and sitting quietly or reading aloud can be equally satisfying for both parties at this stage.

The Final Days

It is normal in these final days and hours for family members or loved ones to share a few moments alone to say their final "good-byes." It is not considered at all unusual to give your loved one "permission" to die, to tell him or her "it is okay to go on."

Your doing so will not hasten death, but rather it is considered a powerful time for you and your loved one to acknowledge the time is near. A tearful and emotionally difficult time for everyone, this "permission" starts each of us down the road to the final grieving process. It is believed to make the passage easier for the person dying and may be a moment you hold forever dear in your heart.

Your loved one may not appear interested in wanting food or drink. It is common to see a decreased need for food and drink as the body no longer desires or requires nutrition and hydration. The digestive system in the body is starting to slow down and the person may not be interested in food. Because the digestive system is slowing down, the body is not absorbing or using calories.

Accept that the decreased appetite is a normal function at this stage and avoid trying to force someone to eat. It is not unusual, however, for the person to suddenly request a favorite meal after not eating for days.

Your loved one may exhibit an increase in restlessness. He or she may pull at the pajamas or bed covers. The restlessness is related to a slowing of the body's circulation. You may actually witness leg tremors or jumping and twitching muscles. This occurs because the body is starting to withdraw blood and oxygen from the limbs. The body functions are starting to slow down.

Do not try to force food in a person as you increase the risk of choking to death. The body is doing what it needs to do. Even placing feeding tubes in a person will not stop death. The body is preparing to cease its function.

At this point, the body is starting to withdraw circulation from the limbs and is focusing on circulation in the trunk or core of the body. Kidneys, liver, lung and heart function are still viable, but the body is starting to slow down. At this point you may also see a slowing of breathing and pulse.

Make certain the person is turned and repositioned every two hours to avoid the development of pressure ulcers (also called bedsores). Because of the body's slowing circulation, the person can rapidly develop these wounds. You can use pillows to elevate legs and hold the person on his/her side when you turn him/her. Keep an additional pillow to place between the legs/knees to help him/her stay comfortable when he/she is lying on their side.

Your loved one may have difficulty swallowing. Try offering semi-liquids such as broths or thin soups in small amounts and at frequent intervals. These can be easier to swallow. Make certain your loved one's head is elevated, either by raising the bed or by using pillows.

Remember that as your loved gets closer to death, you will be more focused on making certain his or her mouth is kept moist by using a medical toothbrush/sponge. Always tell the person you are now giving him/her a sip of water or use a straw to help her receive liquids.

The Final Hours

When death is close, your loved one will now begin to exhibit signs that the end of life is very near. The following symptoms indicate death is days or hours away.

Your loved one may begin to experience a fever that appears to come and go, followed by a general clamminess. As the body goes through the process of shutting down and kidney and liver function slow, the body becomes overwhelmed by infection. As a response, the body raises its temperature to fight the infection, one last effort at life. Antibiotics will not serve in this instance as the body is close to death and organ function is ceasing.

Your loved one may not respond to sound or speech. No one is certain whether the person can hear and understand what is happening around him/her during this time. Nonetheless, we speak to the person as though he/she can still hear. Many people believe even if their loved one cannot hear sound physically, perhaps they can hear spiritually.

Your loved one may not appear to visually respond to you. As the activity of the brain slows in preparation for death, so do the actions and functions of the brain. The eyes response to light is considered a lower brain function and so the brain doesn't expend final energy towards vision.

Your loved one may not follow movement around the room or appear aware of new persons entering or exiting the room. The eyes may have a different look to them, not as bright and alert for example and may become fixed in one area. This fixation is called "dolls' eyes."

Your loved one may exhibit trembling or twitching in his/her legs and arms. This is known as "pre-termination agitation." As blood circulation continues to slow, the muscle cells react to the loss of oxygen by constricting. This is also a sign that death is close.

Your loved one may now begin to exhibit a gurgling sound in his/her throat. This is also known as the death gurgle. It means the body is no longer using energy to swallow and saliva is pooling in the back of the throat. These secretions cannot be suctioned, but medications are available which will help dry them up. This can be difficult for some families to listen too, but remember it is a normal phase. There is also an increase in blood acidity as heart function, circulation and organ function are changing. This acidity is linked to the gurgling.

Keep the head elevated, either through pillows or by raising the bed. Use water now to keep the mouth moist and use the toothbrush/sponge to keep the tongue clean and the mouth free of mucus build-up.

Your loved one will probably be semi-comatose at this stage, but when cleaning the mouth or swabbing the teeth and tongue, continue to tell him or her what you are doing.

The gurgling sound also indicates your loved one is now beginning to switch to abdominal breathing. He/she is no longer breathing through his/her nose; so using an oxygen tube at this time is more for the family than the dying person. However, some families choose to do so, as the sound of the machine can mask the sound of the gurgling.

You can tell your loved one is breathing abdominally by observing him/her. The chest is no longer rising up and out with each breath, instead the stomach area below the rib cage is rising with each breath. The mouth is now open continuously as the person has switched from nose breathing to mouth and abdominal breathing.

The jaw is relaxed, as the body is no longer using energy to hold the mouth shut. The mouth will stay this way following death.

Your loved one may appear to stop having urine output. This has to do both with a withdrawal from nutrition and hydration and the slow functioning of the kidneys. It is not unusual for the kidneys to greatly decrease function as the body continues slowing organ systems down in preparation for death.

The fingertips and toes may begin to change color and appear bluish or purple. This is due to the continued slowing of circulation. It is also known as mottling. As circulation continues to slow, the calves, knees, buttock, arms and shoulders will often show a coloration change. Some persons may have spontaneous bleeding as the blood clotting mechanisms begin to fail, others may suddenly develop bruising in their muscle tissue.

Bedsores (bed wounds, decubitus ulcers, pressure wounds) can open suddenly, especially in the heels or buttocks. Circulating air mattresses are often used here to make the person more comfortable and reduce the incidence of wounds.

The weight of the sheets on the bed can cause heel wounds to open quickly, so a crate or pillows are used to relieve this weight.

The heart rate, which has been quite rapid, is now slowing. Respiration may drop to 16 and the pulse may drop to 25. Remember not every person will experience this drop in pulse and respiration.

*You may use a blanket or sheet to cover your loved one, but do not use an electric blanket.

*Pain assessment should be done at this point to assure the person's comfort.

The body may begin to develop an odor. As the body is not able to nourish its tissues, necrotic activity begins, meaning the tissue is already dying. This is slight and noticeable only through the scent. This is more common with cancer patients, but can occur with others as well.

You may notice your loved one's eyes are remaining slightly open. This is normal. The person's eyes may stay open after death.

This is unlike what we see on television and you will not be able to pass your hand over the face and close the eyes.

You may now see the breathing pattern change and apnea and/or Cheyne-Stokes breathing, will begin. Death is only hours or even moments away as this point. Apnea means breathing stops for several seconds to 30 seconds or longer. You may think your loved one has died and then he/she will take another breath. At this point you can see the slowing becoming more and more pronounced. At the end, you will see one final breath and your loved one will have passed.

Your loved one may make a loud noise or foam at the mouth in the final breath. This is considered a reflexive action rather than an attempt to communicate. It is not an expression of pain, but instead the last physical expression as breath exits the vocal box and the body. A tiny bit of spittle may also collect at the corners of the mouth and expel during the final breath as well. Again, this is considered a natural occurrence.

Death

Death has now occurred. Your loved one may appear to physically shrink. Commonly, once the essence of life has drawn out of the body, the soul or spirit if you will, the body will present as smaller.

Within minutes, the body will become pale and take on a gray hue. This is because blood cells are loosing oxygen and the blood is starting to pool. The body begins to cool and will no longer feel warm to the touch.

The skin color will lose its glow and its tenacity.

The eyes will be flatter as fluid collects and the light will be gone from them. The eyes may be wide open, slightly open or shut, but most often they will remain open.

The mouth will be open as the jaw is slackened with no muscle message to close the lower jawbone.

The body may or may not have some movement left, very slight, as the final settling of the electrical impulses in the body cease.

The body may release urine or stool as the muscles relax.

Many people at this time feel that the soul is close at hand. It is normal to talk to your loved one, hold her hand, pray and wish her well on the next journey.

It is permissible to request the body be allowed to remain where it is for a couple of hours to allow family to gather and to finish your goodbyes. Some families will request to be allowed to wash or change the body, again a normal act of final loving and kindness. Even though the physical connection has ended, the emotional bond you have shared still remains.

Grief After Death

Despite having gone through the stages of grief a number of times during the dementia process, grief begins anew after death. Until that moment, you could still be with the person you loved. You could hold her hand, brush her hair and rub lotion on her hands. Even with the comfort of spiritual or religious beliefs, death is difficult because the person you loved is physically gone leaving a new void and ache in the lives of those left behind.

While crying and feelings of sadness are a part of grieving when you have lost someone you love to death, whether it was sudden or expected, several other reactions also are a normal part of the grieving process. As mentioned earlier, everyone grieves differently and at different speeds. No one way is correct or better than another. Some people may experience all or several of these symptoms, others may not experience any of them.

- **NUMBNESS**: You may be feeling as though you are on autopilot as the brain has gone into shock. Even if a death was anticipated and you believe you have already grieved or are okay with the loss, your brain is not. The brain turns off in a sense and begins moving memories from present tense to past tense. The brain and body need time to adjust to the loss, so take extra care as you go about your duties. You may find that you are arriving at work or the grocery store but not remembering actually driving there or stopping for red lights. If you find yourself in this situation, let friends drive you or at least take special care to focus on your activities.

- **ANGER**: You may be angry with the person who has died for getting ill or not giving you more time to say good-bye. You may be angry with the caregivers, doctors and hospice personnel who were supposed to help, but seemingly let your loved one die. You may be angry with members of your family or with others around you because you feel they don't understand your pain or do not appear to be grieving appropriately. You may be angry with God. Anger is a normal reaction and will pass in time. Also be aware that others around you may be angry too, so try to be tolerant of their actions.

- **REGRETS**: Many people find themselves thinking of all the things they wish they'd done or of all the things they did not do while their loved one was alive. You may experience feelings of regret or guilt that somehow you should have known better or done more or said more or acted differently. Again, these are normal thoughts.

- **FEELING WORSE**: Most people find that it takes almost six weeks before the full effects of grief hit them. It can be a terrible realization to find that you feel even worse after two months than you did after two weeks. This is because in the first few or several weeks, you were experiencing shock. Once the shock passes, you feel begin to feel the pain of loss. This pain likely will continue for months as the body and mind heal. Just remember that you will have better days ahead.

- **PHYSICAL REACTIONS**: You may experience physical pain or more illnesses than usual for the first several months or year after a loved one's death. This is not unusual. You may feel pain in your stomach or chest, experience more frequent colds, feel tired, have difficulty eating and sleeping, or just feel blah. These pains are a real part of the process of grieving.

- **STRANGE SENSATIONS**: You may experience moments when you "see" the deceased in your home or in a crowd or "hear" him/her calling your name. Some people believe this is a memory being played in the mind; others believe the spirit of your loved one is visiting. Having this experience doesn't mean you are going crazy or losing touch with reality. It is simply one of the phenomena reported by many people who have gone through the grieving process.

- **OUTBURSTS**: You may experience sudden tearfulness triggered by something as simple as a commercial or song, or you may feel a sudden rise in anger after hearing an insensitive statement or when seeing a piece of mail addressed to your loved one. You may discover the capacity to be overcome by emotions can continue for months or years after the death. Again, these are normal reactions for some people.

- **SURPRISES**: You may find yourself suddenly surprised that your loved one has died. For example, you may be expecting her to call or knock on the door until you suddenly remember that she has died. Or you may find your self picking up the phone to call her or instinctively driving to her house before remembering, much to your surprise, that she has died. This is more an indicator of a close relationship with the deceased, than a sign that you are behaving abnormally.

- **FORGETFULNESS**: You may easily forget things from telephone numbers to where you put your keys to where you placed the mail. You may notice you are having trouble remembering appointments, birthdays, grocery list items or work tasks. Because your loved one died from Alzheimer's or another dementia, you may even see this as a sign that you have the disease as well. Instead try to remember that your brain is still in shock and you are going through a period of normal grieving. Chances are slim that dementia has suddenly invaded your brain.

- **RECURRING PICTURES**: Some people experience a sensation through which they repeatedly see in their mind disturbing images of their loved one's illness or death. It could feel as if that image is frozen and is the only thought remaining of your loved one. Try instead to replace those images with happier pictures that evoke memories of times with your loved one that brought you joy rather than sadness.

- **DREAMS**: Many people have vivid dreams – both happy and unhappy ones – about their loved one. Some people take comfort in the thought that these dreams are some sort contact from that person or that they are a way of remembering him/her.

Talking to Kids About Dementia and Death

Two of the most common questions I am asked is "How do we tell the grandchildren about Mom's dementia diagnosis/death?" It is estimated we currently have three million teens and pre-teens helping as direct family caregivers in our country alone. Talking to them about what dementia is and what it is doing to their loved one is a critical part of helping them to cope with the burden of care.

Explaining dementia to children is not easy, after all dementia is a terminal disease and obviously affecting someone they love. Here are some tips related to the age of your grandchildren.

PRE-SCHOOL

Do: Just try to keep the information on their level. Young children don't have the ability to process illness and disease or death. This means saying things like "Grannie has a sick brain," or "Sometimes Grannie may not remember your name," or "Grannie has died."

Don't: Try to avoid saying "Grannie is sick" as children can draw inferences from that information. In other words, everybody, including children, gets sick. It is better that the children understand Grannie's behaviors or changes are because of a "sick brain." It helps them begin to make the step to understanding she has a specific illness.

Do: You will probably need to repeat the information several times as younger children live in the "here and now."

Don't: Pretend to know everything. Don't be afraid to admit you may not know all the answers. Children need to feel secure and safe. As long as you can be calm, the kids will probably be okay. Remember, children, even preschoolers, can be quite direct with their questions and they expect answers. Don't make anything up, but try to be honest. Pre-school kids don't need a lot of details; they just need an answer.

Do: Remember it is okay to be sad and to tell this age group you are sad about Grannie's sick brain or her death. Chances are they are already aware people in the family are sad. Talking about it helps them adjust to these new feelings in the family.

Do: Be sure to tell them Grannie's sick brain/death is not their fault. Children, both pre-school and pre-teens, can take on a burden of guilt and feel like their behavior may have caused Grannie's brain to be sick or caused her death.

Do: Be sure to tell them that sometimes a sick brain can make Grannie do things that seem silly or odd. She may forget their names or her manners or say something out of character. Or she may appear to be upset or lost at times. Remind them these things are because of her sick brain and not because of them.

Do: Be aware children can be very literal. They may ask why you can't get in an airplane and go to heaven to get Grannie. They may request a spoon or shovel and want to go get her from the grave. It makes sense to them. If the grave is where she is, then we just need to go get her. Children also have difficulty with the finality of death. They may ask over and over if Grannie is coming back.

Do: Children at this age will grieve and cry. This is a normal reaction for them. As they see adults grieve, so they will grieve as well. But likewise, they may then ask to go outside and play. Remember old age seems like impossibility to them. Just last week, my six-year-old nephew Dos asked a question about death. When I answered him that all living things die, he was incredulous. "You mean I will get old like MeMa one day and then I'll die?" he asked with a look of horror on his face. (MeMa is only 72 and isn't planning on going anywhere anytime soon). But within a few seconds he went on to the next topic – a fellow kindergarten boy had kissed a girl while out on the playground – a scandal no doubt!

SCHOOL AGE AND PRE-TEENS

This age group is quite capable of understanding complex feelings and events, but they will still need your guidance. Their reaction will be very close to your own.

Do: Be prepared for discussions. Eight and nine year old children can process that dementia is a terminal disease and what that means. They can understand illness and death. They may ask detailed questions about the disease progression. And because they are more likely to have a literal thinking process, they may ask painfully frank questions. "Is Grannie going to die?" "Does she hate me?" "Is she sick because I was bad?"

Do: Watch for signs they are suffering emotionally and physically. Stomach aches, headaches, withdrawn or depressed behavior, strange aches and pains, or bad dreams are not uncommon. Let the teacher know about Grannie if schoolwork suffers or seek additional support for your child.

Don't: Pretending nothing is wrong when the children are around can have serious negative impacts on them. Dementia and death affect the family cycle and its dynamics. Keeping information secret can lead children to believe they are somehow responsible for changes.

Do: Support them in their grief. They will be sad not only for their loss, but also because you are grieving. And remember, this person had value to them too. Their feelings will closely mimic your own.

TEENAGERS

This can be a challenging group. A child that has been very close to his grandmother may withdraw or be easily hurt by changes in her behavior or appearance. At times, teenagers may appear uncaring or refuse to visit. The perception of appearing not to care may be related more to what is occurring with the teenager -- school, hormones, physical changes, etc. Or the teenager may be overwhelmed at the thought of losing Grannie or seeing declines and changes in Grannie's abilities.

Teenagers can also be easily embarrassed. They may be afraid of experiencing or exhibiting emotion about Grannie's dementia or death. They may be unable to talk about their feelings or fears.

Do: Offer to be available to talk about what is happening to Grannie.

Don't: Trying to force teenagers to respond may only push them farther away.

Do: Allow teenagers time to adjust to the announcement of Grannie's dementia or death.

Don't: Everyone gets frustrated. Some people experience this as anger. Don't tell your teenager to stop having his/her feelings. After all, a dementia diagnosis or death of a loved one starts the process of grieving and remember, all of us, regardless of our age, grieve differently. The death of a beloved grandparent will most likely be the first death a child remembers, so this can be especially difficult.

Do: Teenagers grieve differently. Try to understand his/her feelings when your teen returns from the funeral service and wants to go to the movies or be with friends. Again, the thought of old age is almost beyond their ability. After all, nothing in their body hurts yet, hair loss and wrinkles are not a challenge, and his/her whole life is in front of them.

Grief, Bereavement and Mourning

Grief is the normal reaction we experience following the death of a loved one. It can manifest itself in several ways. One way is a physical reaction. This could be experienced by an increase or decrease in one's appetite, headaches, stomach aches, hypersomnia or insomnia, illness, or physical aches and pains which cannot be explained, etc. Some people might also experience a mental reaction such as anger, feelings of guilt or remorse, depression, sadness and anguish.

Emotional reactions such as anger, guilt, lashing out, inappropriate responses to situations or others is another type of reaction you could experience. The last type is a social reaction. This might feel like an overwhelming sensation when you see a person or persons who remind you of your loss, when you return to work or the routine you had before the death, or when you are in a place you might have been with your loved one, like church, a favorite restaurant or the grocery store.

Bereavement is the period of time after the death occurs. Grief is beginning to be experienced and the process of mourning your loved one has begun. This period starts following death and before the funeral, but the time can vary from person to person. The variation is based on your age, emotional maturity, the amount of time spent anticipating the loss of your loved one and how close you were to your loved one.

There are generally four phases of bereavement: disbelief and shock, that is a general numbness as the brain struggles to process the information of death and begins shifting memory from present to past, a searching sensation as you attempt to find the person (you may even "see" your loved one in the home or in a crowd), disorganization as you struggle to make sense of your world without your loved one and reorganization as you begin to readjust to your world.

Mourning is the process in which you adapt to the death of your loved one. Society's culture, mores, rules, rituals and customs dictate how we grieve, how long we grieve or whether we receive support from others while we grieve.

Last Notes and Thoughts

David Kessler, a student of Kubler-Ross and a scholar of the dying process, has a wonderful passage in his book **The Needs of the Dying.** To paraphrase him, he writes that in the moment of a person's birth, loved ones were reaching for that new soul. A mother, a father, a grandparent, aunt, uncle, sibling, all eagerly reaching to welcome that new person to our world.

Why, Kessler asks, is it then so hard for us to believe that in that moment of death, those same souls are not once again reaching for their loved one? The journey hasn't ended and your loved one is not alone.

I find Kessler's words to be so comforting, but I can't speak to a person's internal thoughts or beliefs of life or life after death.

In my career I have known only one person who believed there was nothing after death. His wife's decline and death was particularly difficult for him because he had no beliefs.

I can't tell you what's right or wrong. I can only share with you events I have seen that have had a profound effect on my life. I have no explanation, other than that there is a higher power. There is something there. Now I can't give you faith, but I can give you a few stories.

Robert's Story

Robert had been brought by his family to the dementia community I oversaw in Virginia. As his family decorated his room with pictures his young grandchildren had drawn, his children took turns sitting with him.

An old man, well into his late eighties, Robert slipped further and further into the final time of life and remained unresponsive to his family's presence.

Suddenly one day he sat up in bed. Pointing to the ceiling, above his bed he loudly declared "No! No I tell you, I'm not ready!"

His son jumped and grabbing his father's hand asked him what was wrong.

"That lady, that lady there," he said, pointing back at the ceiling. "She says it is time to go, but I'm not ready."

Indeed, Robert wasn't ready. One lone child had not yet arrived from California. She wasn't due for another three days. Robert died in the morning, one day after his last child came to say "goodbye."

⌣

Patricia's Story

Patricia and Jay had fallen in love as teenagers. Through Jay's military career and deployment to Vietnam and the Far East and finally back to the states, Pat had raised their children and greeted each day with an exuberance and joy.

A woman who loved life, Jay's feisty "Boston Babe" had slowly succumbed to dementia. After more than a decade of struggling with the disease, suddenly, within just a year's time, she had gone from Stage Five to Stage Seven and death's door. This final part of dementia, a time that usually runs for years, had taken only months. And in those few months Pat lost her ability to walk, eat, or speak.

But she still responded to her beloved Jay. At breakfast, lunch and dinner, he came faithfully. Encouraging another bite of food, holding her hand and walking her down the hallway, putting her favorite lotion on her hands. Finally, he could only push her wheelchair down the hallway. Sitting with her in the evening, his deep soothing voice seemed to calm her to peaceful sleep.

As quickly as she had progressed to the end of dementia, she begin to fail in the early morning. With a frantic phone call, I woke Jay to the news Pat was leaving us quickly. Within 10 minutes, Jay was running down the hall to Pat's room. And in that final moment, in that final breath, this woman, who hadn't spoken in weeks, spoke. With only one word, she defined how little we know about dementia and true love. With her dying breath, Pat called her beloved's name. "Jay."

Caroline's Story

Caroline had raised her two sons, on her own, a single mom. In the process, she graduated college and rose through the ranks of a state agency. After the boys had grown, left and started their own families, love found her. She retired, married the love of her life and moved to a ranch. A spiritual woman, Caroline told me she found her faith stronger than ever.

But one day, her husband, a farmer and rancher, didn't come back to the house for lunch. Caroline's search found him crushed under the tractor, her beloved Bill gone. A few days later, at his funeral, she collapsed with a blinding pain in her head.

The MRI confirmed a large tumor, non-operable. Suddenly, her ranch was gone, her cattle sold, even her dog was given away and she found herself back in Austin with full-time caregivers helping her perform basic tasks and self care.

As death drew closer, I visited Caroline one last time. Her sons had been called and they were on their way. Her eyes half-open, her breathing shallow and abdominal, she was semi-comatose and unaware of my presence.

Caroline had a family Bible in her bedroom, but it was so worn, I didn't want to disturb it. Instead I picked up a new Bible her friend had left. I talked as though she could hear me. "Caroline, I'll read to you while we wait."

As I had so often before when someone lies dying, I read Psalms 23-25, the Christmas story and the Easter story aloud. My thinking is people like Caroline had heard these stories throughout her life; from the time she was born. The least I could do for her was read them to her one last time.

Through it all, Caroline never moved, her eyes never blinked. Finally I told her I would read one last passage, from whatever page the Bible opened to. I had never done this before, but

Caroline's sons hadn't arrived and I knew she had missed being able to attend her church in the country.

I held the Bible in the palm of my right hand and it fell open to Ecclesiastes 3.

"To every thing there is a season, and a time to every purpose under the heaven: A time to be born, and a time to die; a time to plant, and a time to pluck up that which is planted; A time to kill, and a time to heal; a time to break down, and a time to build up; A time to weep, and a time to laugh; a time to mourn, and a time to dance; A time to cast away stones, and a time to gather stones together; a time to embrace, and a time to refrain from embracing; A time to get, and a time to lose; a time to keep, and a time to cast away; A time to rend, and a time to sew; a time to keep silence, and a time to speak; A time to love, and a time to hate; a time of war, and a time of peace…"

Caroline's sons arrived a short time later and they held their mother's hands as she died. A few days later I was at her funeral. The pastor finished his eulogy and then asked everyone to open their Bibles and read along with him for Caroline's favorite passage – Ecclesiastes 3.

Lillian's Story

*I*was speaking in Midland, Texas one day and afterwards a woman approached me. She shared a story about her husband's dementia and his death.

Married 57 years, her beloved James had developed Alzheimer's. As the disease had progressed, she had been forced to place James in a skilled facility. Lillian visited frequently, but the drive to the nursing home from their ranch was several hours and meant she had could only come every other day.

At the end of each visit, Lillian would say to James "I love you as big as the sky!" Throughout their marriage James would always reply "A sky as blue as your eyes." But because of the dementia, he had not spoken a word or sentence in several months.

That evening, as she prepared to leave, Lillian kissed his cheek again and said "I love you as big as the sky!" And James replied "A sky as blue as your eyes." James died in his sleep that night, his final words given to the woman he loved.

Jay's Story

*I*t is fitting that "Pat's Story" preceded this. As I was finishing this revision, I received a call from Jay and Pat's son Mike that Jay had died. Jay had become a dear friend during Pat's illness and following her death. We often had dinners together and when our dogs had puppies, Jay took the pick of the litter. He called the puppy "Babe" in honor of his beloved Pat.

Even when I moved across the country, Jay and I spoke every two weeks and on holidays. He would ask about the drought in Texas, inquire if I was keeping my car clean, and laugh about his pristine white Toyota Camry with the personalized license plate – Jay & Pat.

In the years after Pat's death, Jay never stopped grieving for or missing his wife. She was always on his mind and he looked forward to the day he would see her again, as that was his faith.

Returning from Jay's funeral in Arlington, I was thinking about Pat and Jay and the time I was injured in Marion, Virginia. A shattered ankle meant I couldn't drive back to Texas and without hesitating Jay sent his car and his son Mike to transport me home. I was passing Marion just then, the roadside park that was the site of the ankle accident and thinking about Jay and Pat and listening to a song by U2. It is the song where Bono is saying he believes in God, but he still questions the afterlife.

As all of these thoughts swirled in my mind, a shiny white car driven by an old white-haired gentleman and his wife suddenly passed me. A shiny white Toyota Camry with the license plates P&J.

At the end of the day, cry when you need to cry. Keep tissues in the car, your purse, your desk at work, next to your favorite chair or bed. Understand the process takes years, not days, and it is okay to grieve.

To learn more about death and the dying process, try these books:

How We Die, Reflections on Life's Final Chapters, Sherwin B. Nuland, M.D.

The Needs of the Dying, A Guide for Bringing Hope, Comfort and Love to Life's Final Chapter, David Kessler.

To learn more about dementia read:

Everything You Wanted to Know About Memory But Forgot to Ask, Ronald Devere, M.D.

For other thoughts about life and death, try these books:

Many Lives, Many Masters, Brian L. Weiss, M.D.

One Last Time, John Edward.

To learn more about how most of us will age read:

The Mature Mind and **The Creative Mind,** Gene Cohen, M.D.

My thoughts and prayers are with each of you and your loved ones. Please feel free to contact me if I may be of any additional assistance.

I can be reached anytime via my website. Go to www.tamcummings.com and I will gladly respond to any questions you might have.

Take care of yourself.

Tam

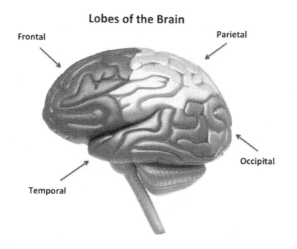

Lobes of the Brain

Frontal   Parietal

Occipital

Temporal

The **Frontal Lobes** are responsible for: Abstract Thought, Attention, Behavior, Coordination of Movement, Creative Thought, Imagination, Impulse Control, Inhibition, Initiative, Intellect, Judgment, Memory, Problem Solving, Producing and Understanding Language, Rational Thought, Reflection, Speech and Some Emotions.

The **Temporal Lobes** are responsible for: Auditory Memories, Cursing, Fear, Hearing, Language, Music, your Sense of Identity, Singing, Some Behavior and Emotion, Smell, Some Visual Pathways, Speech and Visual Memories (faces, places, foods, objects).

The **Occipital Lobes** are responsible for: Depth Perception, Reading, Visual Acuity, Facial Recognition and Vision.

The **Parietal Lobes** are responsible for: Appreciation of Form through Touch, Body's Temperature Perception, Sensory Combination and Comprehension. Some Language and Reading Functions, Some Visual Functions, Taste and Touch.

Made in the USA
Monee, IL
21 September 2020

43099478R10203